W9-BDK-269

FOREVER FAT LOSS

ESCAPE THE LOW CALORIE AND LOW CARB DIET TRAPS AND ACHIEVE EFFORTLESS AND PERMANENT FAT LOSS BY WORKING WITH YOUR BIOLOGY INSTEAD OF AGAINST IT

BY: ARI WHITTEN

www.ariwhitten.com

Copyright © 2015 Ari Whitten

Publishing services provided by **Archangel Ink**

ISBN: 1942761635
ISBN-13: 978-1-942761-63-1

Table of Contents

Introduction

Have you ever gone on a fat loss diet and exercise program and experienced an initial period of weight loss, but then, for some strange reason, over the next year or so you slowly regained back all the weight you lost?

Maybe you've even been in this cycle for the last 5 or 10 years—losing and regaining the same 5, 10, or 20 pounds over and over again. Or maybe all your years of dieting and fat loss exercise programs have just led you into a state where you now bust your butt in the gym multiple times per week and eat hardly anything, yet you are *still* seeing no fat loss.

Diet after diet, and exercise program after exercise program, and nothing but years of spinning your wheels to show for it.

All those diets do seem to work initially, right? When you were counting those calories, or when you were on that low-fat or low-carb diet, you probably did lose lots of weight. But then for some reason, you slowly just seemed to have a harder and harder time sticking to the program. In hindsight, maybe you thought afterwards:

"I just failed to keep the weight off because I didn't stick with the program—I cheated with my diet and I didn't stick to the exercise program like I was supposed to. I took too many days off. I ate too many calories or too many carbs. If I just had a little more willpower, I could have stuck to the diet and exercise program, and I would be lean right now."

During the last half century where we have witnessed both the obesity epidemic and the rise of the fat loss industry, this is the conversation that tens of millions of overweight people have had in their heads.

Millions of fat people in search of weight loss have been told by all the fitness and nutrition authorities that the solution is very simple: "Eat fewer calories, and burn more calories."

We've all heard the calories in, calories out concept a thousand times before, and it even seems to make logical sense that everything really is just a simple matter of your conscious decisions around how many calories you eat each day and how many times you go to the gym each week. It makes sense that people are fat just because "they take in more calories than they burn," and to lose fat, they just need to "take in *less* than they burn."

In fact, for over a decade, I was one of those people preaching to all of my training and nutrition clients that "eat less and burn more" was the answer to fat loss. And regretfully, I even occasionally came down hard on clients who had regained some weight for their inability to "stick to the program." Whenever their fat loss efforts stalled, my answer was always:

"Fat loss isn't rocket science. If you're overweight, it can only be because of two possible things—you're either not burning enough calories or you're eating too many. Period. To fix this, you simply need to eat less and burn more. End of story."

Pretty much every trainer, nutritionist, and weight loss physician tells us that it really is this simple, and we believe it. After all, when we're getting inundated with that message from every magazine, article, book, and TV show, how could we possibly think otherwise?

According to this view, the problem—the reason that so many people fail to achieve lasting fat loss—is simply people's inability to stick to their diet and exercise programs. Maybe if we had trainers and nutritionists holding these people accountable and making sure that they really stick to their diet and exercise program, they would get lasting results. Case in point: *The Biggest Loser* TV show. Here we can clearly see what happens when people implement a diet and exercise program where they have professional guidance from trainers and nutritionists making sure they do things right, and making sure that they stick to their calorie deprivation programs. And without a doubt, it works like a charm—these people often lose 50, 75, or even 100 pounds or more.

So the problem of fat loss has been forever solved! It's as simple as eating fewer calories and burning more. You just need to have the willpower to stick to the program. Case closed.

Or wait, perhaps I spoke a bit too soon...

As it turns out, over 90% of *Biggest Loser* participants regain all the weight they initially lose! [1] [2]

When we look at the scientific studies on deliberate calorie deprivation in the general population, we find the same thing: Over 95% of people who use this approach *fail* to achieve lasting fat loss! For some strange reason, virtually every study conducted on the subject over the last 60 years has shown that when people try to lose weight by intentionally taking in fewer calories than they're burning, they almost always exhibit a pattern of initial weight loss followed by complete fat regain in the next several months or years. In fact, studies now show that a huge percentage of people are actually *fatter* two years after beginning a diet and exercise program than they were before it![3]

---

1 Johannsen, D. L., Knuth, N. D., Huizenga, R., Rood, J. C., Ravussin, E. & Hall, K. D. (2012). Metabolic slowing with massive weigh loss despite preservation of fat-free mass. J of Clin Endocrinology & Metabolism, 97(7). doi: 10.1210/jc.2012-1444.

2 Dulloo, A.G & Girardier, L. (1990). Adaptive changes in energy expenditure during refeeding following low-calorie intake: evidence for a specific metabolic component favoring fat storage. Am J Clin Nutr. 52(3), 415-420.

3 Dieting Does Not Work, UCLA Researchers Report. Retrieved from: http://newsroom.ucla.edu/releases/Dieting-Does-Not-Work-UCLA-Researchers-7832?RelNum=7832

It's important to point out that this failure to achieve lasting fat loss is *not* because they gave up on their diet and exercise programs—most of these people *continue* to try to diet and exercise. They are failing because their biology is not allowing them to stick to the program—their hunger pangs and cravings become too much to fight, and eventually they are forced to give in.

The strange reality is that although every authority is telling us that "eating less and burning more" is the path to fat loss (just like I did for so many years), virtually everyone who tries this approach fails to achieve that in the long term.

And when you inevitably fail, you are put in a very peculiar position: You failed doing the thing that everyone tells you is the right thing to do, so all that you can do is feel defeated and hopeless, and blame yourself with all the "I should've stuck to the program...I should've done this or that" type of self-flagellation.

What I'm going to show you in this book is something extremely important: **It's *not* your fault!**

You haven't failed because of your lack of willpower to stick to your calorie restriction and calorie burning program. You failed because the program *failed you!* The fitness and nutrition industry failed you. The calories-in, calories-out paradigm has failed you. Those preaching that the solution to fat loss is simply "eat less and burn more" have failed you.

I was wrong. And everyone else who thinks the answer to fat loss is as simple as eating less calories and doing more exercise is wrong, too.

What you're about to discover in this book is a revolutionary paradigm shift and a quantum leap forward in how we approach fat loss.

This paradigm shift can be summed up very simply:

Fat Loss Isn't About Willpower and Starvation—It's About *Biology!*

This book is going to show you that the only intelligent approach to fat loss is to *work with* your biology instead of against it.

This is a radical new way of approaching fat loss completely unlike all the low-calorie, low-fat and low-carb diets you've seen before. What you're about to discover is the secret science of lowering your body fat set-point—the secret science of achieving effortless and lasting fat loss.

No more calorie restriction. No more low-carb diets. No more fighting your cravings and suffering through hunger pangs.

Welcome to the new science of effortless and lasting fat loss: *Forever Fat Loss*.

The Gap Between What We Know and What We Do

I don't believe there is any other field of knowledge in existence where there is a bigger discrepancy between what science tells us and what nearly everyone believes, than in the realm of fat loss.

I call it, "The Gap." What is The Gap? Well, The Gap is the mismatch between what we are *doing* in the fat loss industry (what virtually all the trainers, nutritionists, and weight loss physicians are teaching), and what scientists actually *know* about fat loss.

The result of this gap is simple: **Millions of people are pursuing fat loss strategies that science has already proven to be a pathetic failure.**

So why is this going on, and what has created this situation?

Well, I'd like to share a quote from my favorite philosopher that will help us understand what's going on a little bit more clearly:

"The question 'what shall we do about it?' is only asked by those who do not understand the problem. If a problem can be solved at all, to understand it and to know what to do about it are the same thing. On the other hand, doing something about a problem which you do not understand is like trying to clear away darkness by thrusting it aside with your hands." – Alan Watts

With that said, here's a good description of what's going on in the fat loss industry today—they do not fully understand why people get fat in the first place, and thus, their approach to fat loss is as futile as someone trying to clear away darkness with their hands.

Millions of people are currently pursuing tortuous fat loss strategies that are getting them nowhere except a cycle of losing and regaining the same 20 or 30 pounds. And this is a direct result of our misunderstanding of the true causes of fat gain. Because we don't fully understand the causes of the problem we're trying to fix, our approach to fat loss is flawed from the foundation.

In a world filled to the brim with people preaching all sorts of myopic, unscientific, and overly simplistic advice, most people in our society have learned to accept certain "truths" about fat gain and fat loss, which in reality have virtually no scientific support. And, as a result of our incorrect and incomplete understandings of the nature of why people get fat, we are pursuing fat loss strategies that get us nowhere.

I also want to suggest to you that the answer to this situation is in the first part of the above quote—that if you understand a problem accurately, it immediately becomes obvious to you what to do about it. So the solution, in my view, is about understanding the *real* causes of why people get fat in the first place. It's about getting into the nerdy science stuff and creating a *complete* understanding of why we get fat, rather than continuing to oversimplify things and to operate in a paradigm created out of that overly reductionistic pseudoscience.

Therein lies The Gap. So where do we go from here?

Well, now we need to get into the science—we need to explore what this gap is all about, why the approach used by the fat loss industry for the last six decades or so has such a high failure rate, and we need to explore what the science is actually telling us about the true causes of fat gain.

Then, I will present a better way—a completely new and revolutionary approach to fat loss rooted in science instead of myth, reductionist physiology, and misinformation. It is not overly complex—in fact, in terms of what you will actually *do* on a practical level, it's mind-blowingly simple and easy. Yet, in terms of the science behind this approach to fat loss, it has taken me about 15 years to figure everything out. What I have developed as a result is a massive shift in paradigm when it comes to fat loss and a radical new scientific approach to achieving lasting fat loss success.

Why the "Eat Less and Burn More" Approach is a Failure for Long-Term Fat Loss

Virtually every authority on the subject of fat loss tells us that if we want fat loss, it's as simple as this: "Eat less and burn more."

Voila! Everything is solved! Well, at least, according to the people who teach this approach.

And it's true—that approach does indeed work to cause fat loss. Well, it works, except for just one very peculiar thing: **Virtually every long-term study conducted on this approach**

shows that it doesn't work for about 95% of people to achieve *lasting* fat loss. 4 5 6 7 8 9 10 11 12 13 14

4 Dokken, B. B., & Tsao, T-S. (2007). The physiology of body weight regulation: are we too efficient for our own good? Diabetes Spectrum, 20(3), 166-170.

5 Johannsen, D. L., Knuth, N. D., Huizenga, R., Rood, J. C., Ravussin, E. & Hall, K. D. (2012). Metabolic slowing with massive weigh loss despite preservation of fat-free mass. J of Clin Endocrinology & Metabolism, 97(7). doi: 10.1210/jc.2012-1444

6 Keesey, R. E., & Hirvonen, M. D. (1997). Body weight set-points: determination and adjustment. J Nutr, 127(9), 91875S-1883S.

7 Freedhoff, Y. (2012, April 26). The biggest loser destroys participant's metabolism. Weighty Matters. Retrieved from http://www.weightymatters.ca/2012/04/biggest-loser-destroys-participants.html

8 Freedhoff, Y. (2013, January 23). When science met the biggest loser. Health. Retrieved from http://health.usnews.com/health-news/blogs/eat-run/2013/01/23/when-science-met-the-biggest-loser

9 Dulloo, A. G., & Girardier, L. (1990). Adaptive changes in energy expenditure during refeeding following low-calorie intake: evidence for a specific metabolic component favoring fat storage. Am J Clin Nutr, 52(3), 415-420.

10 Garner D.M., & Wooley, S. C. (1991). Confronting the failure of behavioral and dietary treatments for obesity. Clinical Psychology, 11, 729–780. doi: 10.1016/0272-7358(91)90128-H.

11 MacLean, P. S., Bergouignan, A., Cornier, M-A., & Jackman, M. R. (2011). Biology's response to dieting: the impetus for weight regain. Am J Physiology - Regulatory, Integrative and Comparative Physiology, 301, R581-R600. doi: 10.1152/ajpregu.00755.2010

12 MacLean, P. S., Higgins, J. A., Jackman, M. R., Johnson, G.C., Fleming-Elder, B. K., Wyatt, H. R., … Melanson, E.L. (2006). Peripheral metabolic responses to prolonged weight reduction that promote rapid, efficient regain in obesity-prone rats. Am J Physiology - Regulatory, Integrative and Comparative Physiology, 29, R1577-R1588. doi: 10.1152/ajpregu.00810.2005

13 Mutch, D. M., Pers, T. H., Temanni, M. R., Pelloux, V., Marquez-Quinones, A., Holst, C., Martinez, J. A., Babalis, D. (2011). A distinct adipose tissue gene expression response to caloric restriction predicts 6-mo weight maintenance in obese subjects1-3. J Clin Nutr, 94(6), 1399-1409. doi: ajcn.110.006858v194/6/1399

In reviewing the studies on dieting and weight loss, Traci Mann notes that short-term weight loss from dieting does occur, but

"... *these losses are* _not maintained_... *It is only the* _rate_ *of weight regain, not the fact of weight regain, that appears open to debate.*"[15]

Here is what the very wise neurobiologist and obesity researcher, Stephan Guyenet has to say on the matter after reviewing all of the studies:

"If there's one thing that's consistent in the medical literature, **it's that telling people to eat fewer calories does not help them lose weight in the long term.**"[16]

Those two quotes pretty much sum up the studies on the effectiveness of calorie restriction in achieving long-term fat loss. Simply put, it doesn't work.

But how could this be? I mean, simple calorie math and thermodynamics should dictate that if a person just eats 500 or 1,000 calories less each day, then he or she should be able to achieve and maintain plenty of fat loss—dozens of pounds of fat could be lost in just 6 months of doing this.

That's not actually what happens, though. As we've already covered, what happens is an initial period of weight loss followed by a slow process of regaining all the fat that was initially lost.

Now at this point, you might be thinking...

"What about exercise? That works for fat loss, right?"

"Well okay, so dieting is not effective for weight loss, but maybe exercise is effective? If I start a program where I burn 500 more calories each day, surely that will result in fat loss. I mean,

14 Sumithran P., & Proietto J. (2013). The defense of body weight: a physiological basis for weight regain after weight loss. Clin Sci (Lond), 124(4), 231-241. doi: 10.1042/CS20120223.

15 Garner DM, Wooley SC. Confronting the failure of behavioral and dietary treatments for obesity. Clin Psychol Rev. 1991;11:729–780. doi: 10.1016/0272-7358(91)90128-H.

16 Guyenet, S. (2010, January 31). The body fat setpoint, part iv: Changing the setpoint. Retrieved from http://wholehealthsource.blogspot.com/2010/01/body-fat-setpoint-part-iv-changing.html

it's simply calorie math—500 calories each day multiplied by seven days a week equals 3,500 calories per week. Three thousand five hundred calories is the amount of calories in one pound of body fat, so...if I burn 3,500 calories each week, I should lose about one pound of fat off my body each week."

Well, it's a nice thought, and much like dieting, it makes sense when analyzed logically on a superficial level. But here's the strange reality of what actually happens:

Despite burning tens of thousands of calories, exercise, as most studies show, does not result in a significant amount of fat loss.

For example, here are a couple of studies done on weight lifting and fat loss:

- Study # 1 - After 6 months of weight lifting, 3 hours per week, they found no fat loss whatsoever.[17]
- Study # 2 – Another study looked at women who got 3 hours a week of personal training for 6 months. They found no significant reduction in fat relative to a control group that spent those 6 months doing nothing.[18]

"Okay, well, maybe weight lifting doesn't result in much fat loss. But surely cardio does!"

As far as "cardio" (the exercise hyped for decades for its supposed "fat burning" ability) is concerned, well, let me share some studies and quotes from researchers on the subject:

17 Church, T. S., Martin, C. K., Thompson, A. M., Earnest, C. P., Mikus, C. R. & Blair, S. N. (2009). Changes in Weight, Waist Circumference and Compensatory Responses with Different Doses of Exercise among Sedentary, Overweight Postmenopausal Women. PLoS ONE 4(2), e4515. oi:10.1371/journal.pone.0004515

18 Willis, L. H., Slentz, C. A., Bateman, L. A., Shields, A. T., Piner, L. W., Bales, C. W., Houmard, J. A. (2012). Effects of aerobic and/or resistance training on body mass and fat mass in overweight or obese adults. J Appl Physiol, 113(12), 1831-7. doi: 10.1152/japplphysiol.01370.2011.

"Despite the popular support for aerobic training, it does not appear to significantly accelerate fat loss, even when combined with a low calorie diet." [19]

Dr. Wayne Miller and colleagues at The George Washington University Medical Centre examined 493 studies carried out on the subject between 1969 and 1994 and found that diet and aerobic exercise provides only a very marginal benefit (in terms of weight loss) when compared to diet alone.

Another 12-week study[20] assigned a group of 91 obese women to one of four groups: Group one followed a restricted calorie diet; group two performed moderate aerobic exercise for 45 minutes for five days each week, and a third group combined the exercise and diet programs. The fourth group acted as controls. Here's what they found:

Method	Weight Loss
Aerobic exercise	1.3kg (2.9lb)
Restricted calorie diet	6.8kg (15lb)
Exercise and diet	7.2kg (15.8lb)

(Note: As previously stated, dieting does indeed result in short-term weight loss, which is why you see the weight loss indicated above. When viewed in the long term, however, virtually all of these people will regain all fat lost from this diet.)

---

19 Finn, C. (n.d). Aerobic exercise: Does it really speed up fat loss?. Retrieved from http://www.timinvermont.com/fitness/aerobic.htm

20 Utter, A.C., Nieman, D.C., Shannonhouse, E.M., Butterworth, D.E., & Nieman, C.N. (1998). Influence of diet and/or exercise on body composition and cardiorespiratory fitness in obese women. International Journal of Sport Nutrition, 8, 213-222.

To put it simply, after doing 45 *hours* of "cardio," they lost less than one pound beyond what they would have if they did no exercise whatsoever!

According to Guyenet: "...Running on a treadmill is not really an effective means to lose body fat if a person is overweight or obese. It's possible that exercise could have a role in preventing obesity, but it's fairly clear from the studies that it's not an effective treatment for obesity." [21]

Here's what exercise scientist Alan Utter has to say on his research into cardio and fat loss: *"Moderate aerobic exercise training has a minor, non-significant effect on fat mass."*[22]

Even well-known trainer and nutritionist John Berardi acknowledges that exercise alone—even extremely well-designed exercise programs facilitated by professional trainers—have negligible effects on body fat.[23]

In summation, if you just add an exercise routine into your life to burn more calories, you can do *months* of exercise and burn 50,000 calories in total—which, based on simple calorie math, should result in about 14 pounds of fat loss (50,000 calories/3,500 calories per pound of fat = 14.2 pounds of body fat). Yet, after burning those 50,000 calories, most studies indicate that you might hope to lose two or three pounds at best, or, in many cases, none at all.

What About Diet And Exercise Together?

At this point, you might be thinking, "Okay, well dieting may not be effective. And exercise may not be effective. But what

---

21 Kresser, C. (2010). Episode 1 – Stephan Guyenet on causes and treatment of obesity. Podcast retrieved from http://chriskresser.com/podcast-episode-i-interview-with-stephan-guyenet-on-obesity-and-weight-loss

22 Utter, A.C., Nieman, D.C., Shannonhouse, E.M., Butterworth, D.E., & Nieman, C.N. (1998). Influence of diet and/or exercise on body composition and cardiorespiratory fitness in obese women. International Journal of Sport Nutrition, 8, 213-222.

23 Berardi, J. When exercise doesn't work. Retrieved from: http://www.precisionnutrition.com/when-exercise-doesnt-work

about combining diet and exercise both simultaneously? That has to work, right? I mean, I've seen the Biggest Loser TV show where everyone loses 50, 75, or even 100 pounds from doing both diet and exercise together."

It is true—restricting calorie intake in conjunction with added exercise does indeed result in plenty of weight loss. This is an undeniable and undebatable fact. If you do lots of exercise in conjunction with starving your body of calories for weeks or months (if you are able to deal with those tortuous hunger pangs, that is), you absolutely will lose lots of weight—just like the participants of The Biggest Loser do.

But like I told you before, the latest research indicates that over 90% of Biggest Loser participants gain back all the weight they lose after the show is over.[24] And dozens of other studies have shown similar figures for the general population[25]— so this is nothing unique to the Biggest Loser, this is an epidemic throughout the weight loss industry. People are achieving massive short-term fat loss success of 50 or even 100 pounds, but something is happening to cause people to regain all the fat they lose. The study on Biggest Loser participants found that it was not due to them failing to try to continue to exercise and follow their diet, but that it was due to "metabolic adaptation." They found that the participants were actually burning hundreds of calories less per day than when they were obese and sedentary! Even beyond the normal reduction in calorie burning that accompanies weight loss, these participants were found to be burning *over 500 calories less per day* than would be predicted based

---

24 Freedhoff, Y. (2012, April 26). The Biggest Loser destroys participants' metabolisms. Retrieved from http://www.weightymatters.ca/2012/04/biggest-loser-destroys-participants.html

25 Dulloo, A.G & Girardier, L. (1990). Adaptive changes in energy expenditure during refeeding following low-calorie intake: evidence for a specific metabolic component favoring fat storage. Am J Clin Nutr. 52(3), 415-420.

on their body mass.[26] That is, their metabolisms slowed down to a sloth's pace. And guess what a slow metabolism does? It predisposes to regaining fat very easily.

Any way you look at it—whether diet alone, exercise alone, or diet and exercise combined—the long-term results are undeniably pathetic.

Why is this metabolic adaptation happening? Why doesn't burning 50,000 calories with cardio result in 14 or 15 pounds of weight loss? Why doesn't restricting calorie intake by 500 or 1,000 calories below what you're eating now result in you attaining lasting fat loss of 50 or 100 pounds—like simple calorie math would suggest?

---

26 Freedhoff, Y. (2012, April 26). The Biggest Loser destroys participants' metabolisms. Retrieved from http://www.weightymatters.ca/2012/04/biggest-loser-destroys-participants.html

Most People Think That If You Have a Calorie Deficit, Your Body Is Forced to Burn Off Body Fat. Wrong! Here's What Really Happens...

The leaders of the fat loss industry preach that "the first law of thermodynamics says 'energy cannot be created or destroyed,' so that means that fat loss is just simple calorie math—if we restrict calorie intake below what we burn, then our body is forced to burn off all our body fat! It has to get that energy from somewhere, and that somewhere is body fat."

But in actuality, the first law of thermodynamics only says: "If you are taking in fewer calories than you burn, your body must respond to that situation by *doing something* to eliminate that deficit of energy—perhaps by burning off your body fat, or perhaps through something else." It is indeed true that energy can neither be created nor destroyed, but what is not true is that if you restrict calories below what you burn, your body simply responds by burning off body fat and making you lean.

In reality, what the studies show very clearly is this: When you restrict calorie intake below what you burn, you will initially lose weight, but then *something* happens (even when you are sticking to the diet/exercise program) that causes weight loss to come to a grinding halt, and then causes you to slowly gain back all the weight you initially lost. Something out of your control is happening that causes you to fail.

So what is that something?

Metabolism slowdown!

To be more accurate, being in a calorie deficit results in three main metabolic adaptations:

1. It decreases thyroid hormone, the main controller of metabolic rate. Less thyroid hormone means decreased calories out from decreased basal metabolic rate.

2. It destroys muscle—as much or more muscle in many cases, than fat—in order to further decrease calorie burning. Muscle tissue is more active than fat, so by preferentially destroying muscle rather than fat tissue, it can lower the body's calorie burning far more.

3. It causes fatigue. Now, fatigue does a few interesting things: First, it decreases your desire and ability to perform exercise (that means decreased calories out); it decreases your ability to perform during that exercise and push yourself (again, decreased calories out); and even more importantly, it decreases something called NEAT (non-exercise activity thermogenesis), which is the hundreds of calories we typically burn each day involuntarily while twiddling our thumbs, tapping our feet, and through the simple activities of living our life, like walking down the street. Without you even noticing, you start *moving less* throughout the day, and your body ends up burning hundreds of calories less than it would normally.

These three things are the way that our biology is wired to respond to caloric deficit. This is our body's energy regulation system in action.

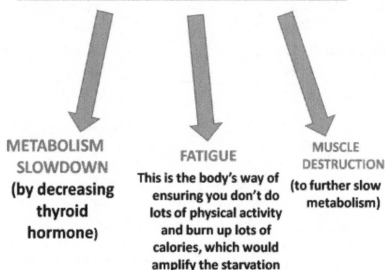

CALORIE DEPRIVATION from diet + exercise

METABOLISM SLOWDOWN (by decreasing thyroid hormone)

FATIGUE
This is the body's way of ensuring you don't do lots of physical activity and burn up lots of calories, which would amplify the starvation

MUSCLE DESTRUCTION (to further slow metabolism)

Through these three simple mechanisms, the body is able to dramatically decrease how many calories it burns each day by many hundreds of calories. And when that happens, no more fat loss.

- This is the *real* reason why we can have people on cardio exercise programs where they burn 50,000 calories—which should theoretically result in almost 15 pounds of fat loss—but often lose less than 3 pounds, or in some studies, none at all.

- This is the *real* reason why we can put people on diets where they are taking in 800 or 1,000 calories less than they normally do (and less than their bodies burn initially) and, a year or two later, find that they are as fat, or *fatter*, than they were when they started the diet.

- This is the *real* reason why, when you combine diet and exercise together like *The Biggest Loser* participants, you get the same thing—lots of weight loss initially, then the body's compensatory mechanisms kick in, and the person regains all the fat they lost.

Bottom line: When the metabolism slows down, fat loss stops. And, what's more, the body actually puts on fat extremely easily, and ultimately causes you to gain back all the weight you initially lost.

Let's look at some specific numbers now. Let's say that you normally take in and burn about 2,000 calories each day, and then you decide to go on a diet and eat only 1,500. Initially, your body will still be burning more than you take in, and you will get weight loss (from a mix of fat and muscle tissue). Then, the body slowly decreases its calorie burning (through decreased metabolism, decreased NEAT, fatigue, and muscle loss) until it's only burning 1,500 calories per day.

Once this happens, it has two very important consequences:

1. Now you're eating much less than you would eat normally, and you're *still* not losing fat.
2. Now it only takes 1,600 or 1,700 calories eaten—*less* than you would normally eat at your maintenance weight—to actually get *fatter!* Before, it would've taken over 2,000 calories, now it only takes over 1,500.

So where do you go from there? Eat even fewer calories? Force yourself to do more exercise, even though you're fatigued and you are already fighting hunger pangs? I don't think so. This is a no-win situation. The only place it leads is a place you don't want to go.

This is the real reason why people fail on the "burn more calories than you take in" program and regain all the fat. It is *not* because it's *your fault*—because you didn't have enough willpower and you failed to stick to your diet and exercise program—it's because you entered into a fight against your own biology, and eventually, your biology won out.

Let me repeat that, because it's worth saying again. If you've been stuck in a cycle of dieting and exercise programs to lose fat, and you've been losing and regaining the same 20 or 30 pounds for years and feeling frustrated and hopeless and like a failure, you need to understand this: **It's not your fault.**

Fat loss isn't about starvation and willpower—it's about biology!

And when you adopt an approach that is built on trying to *fight against* your biology instead of working with it, you will inevitably fail. Fighting against your biology is simply not a fight you can win in the long term. What you will get is short-term weight loss (largely from muscle), followed by metabolic slowdown, and finally, complete and total fat regain.

This simple fact of how our biology is designed to work is what really explains the failure of the "eat less and burn more" approach to fat loss.

But in the face of an absolutely pathetic success rate and an overwhelming amount of scientific evidence to show that "eat less and burn more"—logical as it may seem—doesn't actually work to create sustainable fat loss, what do all the weight loss "gurus" do? They basically pretend like none of the research even exists and go on chanting the mantra "eat fewer calories and burn more"... "eat fewer calories and burn more"... "eat fewer calories and burn more."

Why?

Simple: Because no one has really been able to figure out anything better than that…until now.

The Body Fat Set-Point System: The Secret to Fat Loss

It should now be clear to you that the path to fat loss is *not* through the worn out mantra "eat less and burn more."

If the human body were a machine that just burned 2,000 calories each day no matter what was going on or how much food you were eating, then the calories in/calories out theory would be true and would work perfectly for lasting fat loss. The only problem with the theory is that the human body is not a machine—it is made of dynamic living substance and is always adapting to survive its environment. So when you take in less energy, it adapts for survival very easily by simply *burning less energy*!

As Stephan Guyenet explains: "*... This is where the calories in/calories out theory fails—it doesn't account for this dynamic regulation of energy balance.*"[27]

In other words, the "burn more calories than you take in" approach to fat loss fails to achieve lasting fat loss because the body decreases calorie burning when you take in less calories, in an effort to equalize calories out to the new calories in.

The body is actually fighting against fat loss!

---

27 Kresser, C. (2010). Episode 1 – Stephan Guyenet on causes and treatment of obesity. Podcast retrieved from http://chriskresser.com/podcast-episode-i-interview-with-stephan-guyenet-on-obesity-and-weight-loss

But the real question is *why*? Why is the body doing this? Why would our biology be wired to fight against our efforts to achieve fat loss?

I'll let the very wise neurobiologist and obesity researcher, Stephan Guyenet explain:

"If there's one thing that's consistent in the medical literature, **it's that telling people to eat fewer calories does not help them lose weight in the long term**...Many people who use this strategy see transient fat loss, followed by fat regain and a feeling of defeat. There's a simple reason for it: the body doesn't want to lose weight. It's extremely difficult to fight the fat mass set-point, and the body will use every tool it has to maintain its preferred level of fat: hunger, reduced body temperature, higher muscle efficiency (i.e., less energy is expended for the same movement), lethargy, lowered immune function, *et cetera*." [28]

Ah, the fat mass set-point—a little something that is now understood by every obesity scientist on the planet as the key to fat loss, and something that virtually every trainer, physician, and nutritionist on the planet has never even heard of. (Remember The Gap I keep telling you about?)

What is the fat mass set-point?

It is essentially a biological feedback system that is designed specifically for the purpose of keeping our bodyweight stable over time.

This is the secret key to really understanding fat loss that is completely unknown in a fat loss industry full of people telling you that fat loss is just a simple matter of consciously controlling caloric intake and expenditure with low-calorie diets and exercise.

Once again, I'll defer to Guyenet to explain the crux of what's really going on, since he is one of the world's foremost experts on the body fat set-point system:

---

28 Guyenet, S. (2010, January 31). The body fat setpoint, part iv: Changing the setpoint. Retrieved from http://wholehealthsource.blogspot.com/2010/01/body-fat-setpoint-part-iv-changing.html

"...Fat mass is biologically regulated. So, it's not just the result of conscious decisions to eat less or exercise more or eat more. It's a biologically regulated process ... It has been shown in a number of studies in both animals and humans that if you restrict calories, you can produce fat loss. There's no doubt about that. You also produce a loss of lean body mass. **But as soon as you allow that animal or person to eat as much as they want to eat again, they bounce right back up to their original fat mass.** *And that occurs whether you start with someone who is overweight or someone who is lean.* **So, at least short-term changes in fat mass are compensated for very quickly by the body, and there are a number of mechanisms that are designed to pull fat mass back into the place where the body wants it.***"[29]*

I already explained to you that the calorie deprivation ("burn more than you take in") approach to fat loss fails because of the body decreasing calorie expenditure (metabolism slowdown, etc.). But what I didn't explain to you fully is that this is part of an elaborate system of brain regions and hormones that are *unconsciously regulating our calories in and calories out all the time!*

To put it simply: The "burn more calories than you take in" approach to fat loss fails because it ignores the simple fact that your biology is *wired* to *prevent* you from actually succeeding in burning more calories than you take in for any significant length of time.

Guyenet goes on to say:

"So there's this feedback mechanism that the body has to try to keep fat in a particular place, and that's the reason why just eating less doesn't work, because if you haven't removed the factor that's causing your body to want to store more fat, it's still gonna want to store fat even though you're not giving [it] the calories it needs to continue storing fat, so it's gonna increase hunger, it's gonna decrease metabolic rate, it's gonna increase the efficiency of muscular contractions so your muscles do the same amount of work by expending less energy, decrease body temperature, etc., all of these things designed to pull, as

---

29 http://chriskresser.com/podcast-episode-i-interview-with-stephan-guyenet-on-obesity-and-weight-loss

much as possible, the fat mass back to the place where it wants it. So basically, you can lose fat by eating less, but you'll be fighting yourself. You're fighting your body as long as you haven't changed where the adipostat is set."

This body fat set-point system is fighting our efforts at fat loss and making sure that we gain back all the weight we lose from calorie deprivation.

Now, let me help you understand a little more about what biological regulation of bodyweight actually means and how this whole body fat set-point system actually works.

We already understand this concept in many other aspects of our life, but virtually no one understands that it also applies to fat loss.

In exactly the same way that the body has a built-in system that regulates blood sugar, blood pressure, body temperature, blood oxygen, and sleep/wake cycles, our biology also comes hard-wired with a system designed to regulate our *bodyweight.*

Let me show you what I mean ...

Let's look at three biologically-regulated systems of the body: blood oxygen, sleep/wake cycles, and bodyweight.

First, let's look at oxygen. Let's think about it in exactly the same way that people talk about bodyweight. Let's say you come to me and say, "You know, Ari, I've got this problem I've been dealing with—my blood oxygen is just too high. I need you to help me lower my blood oxygen."

And I say to you, "Oh, if you want to lower the amount of oxygen in your blood, that's really simple! All you have to do is deprive your body of oxygen by holding your breath."

So you hold your breath and, sure enough, it works! You deprive your body of oxygen and your blood oxygen goes down, just like I said it would.

But then what happens?

Well, the body counteracts you holding your breath by first forcing you to breathe, and then hyperventilating to quickly return oxygen levels to normal.

So is lowering the amount of oxygen in your body as simple as just depriving your body of oxygen? Obviously not. You have some conscious control over it—temporarily—but in the end, it is dictated by biology.

Now, let's look at sleep/wake cycles. Let's say you come to me and say, "Ari, look, I have this problem—I'm sleeping too many hours. I sleep, like, eight hours a night, and I just don't have time to sleep that much. I've got work to do and things to get done, and I need more hours that I can be awake working."

I reply: "Oh sure...no problem. There's a really easy solution. All you have to do to decrease the time you're sleeping is just force yourself to stay up until 2 am, set your alarm clock to 4 am, and then force yourself to get up and start your day after only two hours of sleep."

And sure enough, you can do it! You've successfully decreased the amount of sleep you get each night. Voila! Problem solved.

But wait, not so fast...your body then counteracts your sleep deprivation by doing a couple of things. One, it gets really tired so you can't function well. Two, the next night, it will sleep an *excess* to make up for the lost sleep the previous night. Within a few days, the body quickly reestablishes its normal sleep/wake cycle, and you're back to sleeping your normal amount of hours. Again, you have the ability to consciously control things—temporarily—but in the end, it is dictated by biology.

Ok, now let's look at bodyweight, and let's talk about it in exactly the same way as we did with blood oxygen and sleep.

You come to me with your problem: "Ari, look, I have too much fat on my body—I really need to get rid of it."

I reply: "Oh sure, that's no problem at all. There's a really simple solution for that. You see, it's just a problem of taking in too much of the stuff that turns into fat—calories—so you just need to take in less of it."

And sure enough, it works. At least in the beginning.

But then what does the body do? It first increases hunger levels. This motivates you to eat more to cancel out the caloric deprivation. If you are stuck in a famine, and there's no food available, or, more likely in the modern world, you are forcibly restricting your food intake because someone told you that's the best way to get fat loss, then the body will *slow down the metabolism.*

These compensatory responses of the body bring fat loss to a screeching halt, and the slow metabolism (decreased calories out) causes the body to gain weight very easily, *even while eating much less than you normally eat!* So the body quickly regains all the fat that was lost, and bodyweight returns to normal. This is why we see the yo-yo effect, where people continually lose and regain the same 10, 20, or 40 pounds year after year.

	STIMULUS	BODY'S RESPONSE	RESULT
OXYGEN	DEPRIVE YOURSELF OF OXYGEN	HYPERVENTILATION	Blood oxygen returns to normal.
SLEEP	DEPRIVE YOURSELF OF SLEEP	FATIGUE and EXCESS SLEEP	Sleep/wake cycle returns to normal.
BODYWEIGHT	DEPRIVE YOURSELF OF CALORIES	SLOWED METABOLISM (fatigue, decreased NEAT, loss of muscle)	Fat loss stops. All bodyfat that was lost is slowly regained.

Your bodyweight is exactly the same as oxygen and sleep in that it is *biologically regulated.* The only difference is time scale. We can all see this a lot easier on the time scale of oxygen or sleep. It takes only a minute or two to see the body counteract you holding your breath, so it is readily observable. It takes a day or two for the body to counteract sleep deprivation, so it is still readily observable. But with bodyweight, you may lose weight for one month, three months, maybe even six months, and then it may take six months or a year of your body slowly regaining the weight, so it's hard for us to really see what's happening.

And instead of realizing that it's because our body has initiated powerful biological responses that are pulling the fat back on, we instead blame ourselves, thinking it's our failure to stick to the diet or exercise program. The time scale may be different with bodyweight compared to sleep or blood oxygen, but it's exactly the same thing. If you gained all the weight back in two days instead of two months, everyone would immediately see this. It's just harder to see because it's happening over a longer period of time than say, holding your breath or sleeping less.

So how does this system work? How does the body actually regulate our bodyweight?

The way this system works is very complex in terms of all the different hormones and brain regions involved, but in essence, the way the body regulates bodyweight is as simple as this:

The basic way that your body tries to keep a stable bodyweight:

	HUNGER	METABOLISM	RESULT
PERIOD OF OVEREATING	⬇	⬆	Bodyweight stays stable
PERIOD OF UNDEREATING	⬆	⬇	Bodyweight stays stable

To keep bodyweight stable, the body needs to be able to both prevent weight gain from overeating and prevent weight loss from under-eating.

- During a period of over-eating calories, the body responds to that situation by doing two things:

1. Decreasing hunger and
2. Increasing metabolic rate. End result: The body takes in fewer calories and burns more calories and returns you to your normal bodyweight.

- During a period of under-eating, the body does the opposite:

1. Increasing hunger, which is why you will get hunger pangs if you starve your body of calories, and 2) Metabolic adaptations that decrease calorie burning. End result: Body minimizes weight loss and quickly causes you to balloon back up to your normal bodyweight.

Now, why does this happen? Why is the body wired with this body fat set-point system? What is its purpose?

Well, let's think about this in an evolutionary context: Why would our bodies be wired to resist weight loss during a period of calorie deprivation?

Simple: Because having the ability to not starve to death during periods of famine or food shortage is an immensely valuable trait to have if you'd like to survive in an environment where there aren't grocery stores around every corner.

In an article called "The Physiology of Bodyweight Regulation: Are We Too Efficient for Our Own Good?" the scientists concluded that the fat mass set-point evolved because it gave us a survival advantage:

"While losing weight in the short term is achievable, maintaining reduced body weight over the long term has proven to be exceedingly difficult for most people. **At least part of the reason behind the difficulty of maintaining a reduced body weight is the body's ability to activate adaptive mechanisms** that act to minimize weight loss (i.e. the body fat set-point system) ... The ability of an organism to minimize reduction in body weight during long periods of starvation is likely associated with its survival. As a result, millions of years of evolution may have favored organisms with high metabolic efficiency.

It is well documented that, although most people participating in weight-loss programs can successfully lose weight in the short term, the majority of them cannot sustain the reduced body weight in the long run. A plausible hypothesis that can account for the body's tendency to return to its prior weight can be stated as follows: body weight is maintained at a set level, and deviations from the preferred set-point are resisted and minimized by a feedback control system."[30]

In other words, if you were thinking that you'd just restrict calories a little bit and do some more calorie burning exercise and watch your body fat vanish right before your very eyes, well you're in for a big surprise, because the body will fight your fat loss efforts every step of the way. Millions of years of evolution have made sure that your body is *very* good at preventing fat loss.

During times of famine, our ancestors were forced to survive through periods where they were unable to obtain the amount of calories their bodies needed. How did they survive? **By slowing down the metabolism.** (And fatigue, muscle destruction, and decreased NEAT). If you're taking in fewer calories, the body adapts for survival by *burning fewer calories*. The reason is simple. It does this in order to make sure that calories burned do *not* exceed the amount of calories you're taking in.

Of course, there's a certain degree of irony to this whole situation. The very same thing that allowed our species (and all other mammalian species) to survive periods of occasional food

---

30 Dokken, B. B. & Tsao, T. (2007). The physiology of body weight regulation: Are we too efficient for our own good? Diabetes Spectrum, 20, 166-170.

shortage—the reason we are able to exist in the world today—is the very thing that is sabotaging our efforts to achieve fat loss in our modern world of extreme food abundance.

When you put yourself in a perceived famine state by forcibly restricting calories, you are unknowingly fighting a battle against your own biology—a battle that you simply cannot win, and a battle that leads you someplace you don't want to go. As a result, you either end up in a cycle of weight yo-yoing or you train your body into regulating calories at a lower baseline level, where you find yourself eating hardly anything and still not losing any fat. Both of these situations are not very fun.

And every time you fail, you are told to go back and try the "eat less and burn more" approach again, but by now you should know that's not the answer. We'll get to the *real* solution in a minute.

First, there's one more thing about this body fat set-point system that you should understand.

The Fallacy of the Gluttony and Sloth Theory of Fat Gain, and Why We Really Get Fat

So far I've focused on talking about the body fat set-point system through the lens of calorie deficits (famine and dieting), but there is a whole other aspect to this system that's absolutely critical to grasp if you want to understand the true path to effortless fat loss.

Recall the graph I showed you before:

The basic way that your body tries to keep a stable bodyweight:

	HUNGER	METABOLISM	RESULT
PERIOD OF OVEREATING	⬇	⬆	Bodyweight stays stable
PERIOD OF UNDEREATING	⬆	⬇	Bodyweight stays stable

The whole purpose of this system is to keep you at a certain stable bodyweight (your set-point) and to essentially keep you at a healthy, fairly lean bodyweight set-point. It is designed to prevent you from losing too much weight and starving to death during a period of food shortage, *and* to prevent you from getting fat during a period of over-eating. This is an important point: **Our biology is wired by evolution to maintain leanness!**

Think about it: When was the last time you saw a fat lion or wolf or deer or coyote or any other wild animal?

Wild animals are wired with a bodyweight regulation system in exactly the same way that humans are. Fat wild animals do not exist. With the exception of animals preparing for hibernation or animals who live in Arctic regions where large body fat reserves are necessary for survival, the only time an animal doesn't effortlessly maintain a normal, healthy, lean bodyweight is if it's starving to death. This is exactly the same situation we find if we look at wild human populations—and by "wild humans" I mean traditional tribal and hunter-gatherer populations still living out in the forest or desert or jungle. We don't even have to invoke speculative theories based on what our hunter-gatherer ancestors may or may not have been like 100,000 years ago, because we can look at modern tribes living their traditional lifestyle that still exist today, like the Ewe tribe, the Masai, the Kitavans, and numerous others. They, too, have a near-zero incidence of overweight and obesity.

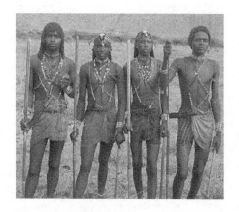
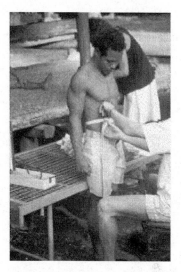

Above: Masai people on the left, and a typical Kitavan on the right.

Obviously, hunter-gatherers and wild animals don't even know what a calorie is, let alone have to consciously monitor their food intake and energy expenditure all the time in order to stay lean. They stay lean *effortlessly* without ever having a single thought around restricting or burning calories.

This is critically important to understand: <u>The *normal* and natural state of the body is to be lean, and when you are living in congruence with your genome, you stay *effortlessly* lean.</u>

If you understand everything we've gone over so far—that you have this system built into your biology that's designed to regulate your bodyweight—then there is one very important question you should now be asking...

"If we have this system to regulate our bodyweight, then how does anyone get fat in the first place?!"

Great question!

This brings me back to the quote I shared with you at the beginning of this book:

"If a problem can be solved at all, to understand it and to know what to do about it are the same thing. On the other hand, doing something about a problem which you do not understand is like trying to clear away darkness by thrusting it aside with your hands."

Understanding the problem—figuring out how anyone gets fat in the first place—is the absolute most important thing we need to do if we want to be successful in achieving fat loss. And this is exactly the issue with the fat loss industry—it does *not* fully understand the true causes of fat gain, and thus its approach to solving that problem is destined for futility.

Let me show you The Gap—this mismatch between how the fat loss industry understands how people get fat, and how obesity scientists now understand it.

Take a look at the graph below.

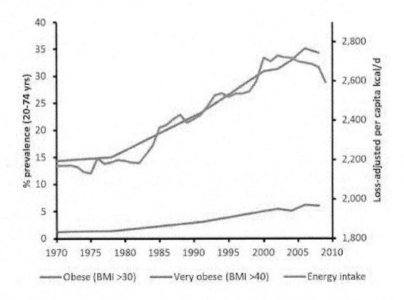

In the graph above, you'll notice that over the last 45 years, calories consumed have gone up by about 400 calories per day per person. This is a simple and undeniable fact. And just as undeniable is the fact that the obesity epidemic has coincided perfectly with this increase in calorie consumption.

Both the people in the fat loss industry and the obesity scientists agree on these two basic facts. However, we see a big gap between the two groups in the *interpretation* of this data.

The Fat Loss Industry's Interpretation: People in the fat loss industry look at this data and say, "Well, there's the cause of fat gain right there! It's obvious. We're eating more calories, and we've gotten fatter. The lines even mirror each other perfectly— we have gotten fat in direct proportion to how many calories we're consuming. The reason that we're fatter today than we were 40 or 50 years ago is simply that we're eating more calories than we used to" That way of understanding the obesity epidemic is known as the "Gluttony and Sloth Theory of Obesity." The problem according to this theory (and according to virtually everyone in the fat loss industry) is that we're simply consuming too many calories due to gluttony and sloth. You know, we're lazy couch potatoes and we have no self-control around our eating habits; therefore, we eat too many calories and get fat.

This is logical and appears to make sense on the surface—if you eat more calories, then, of course, you'll be fatter. It's as simple as that, right?

Oh, except for one little thing. Humans, like all other mammals, have maintained leanness effortlessly for hundreds of thousands of years. In other words, that squiggly line of calorie consumption has basically been flat for tens of thousands of years—basically all of human history. But all of the sudden, about 50 years ago, that line began to go up. And when that happened, we began to get fat.

That is the reason that scientists have a fundamentally different paradigm of fat gain than the fat-loss industry.

Obesity Scientists' Interpretation: Scientists do not subscribe to the gluttony and sloth theory. Instead of framing the issue as simple calorie math, scientists ask the simple question: **Why? Why are we eating more calories?** What all of the sudden changed that made humans go from effortlessly regulating a lean bodyweight (without even knowing what a calorie was) to eating hundreds of calories more per day and becoming fat? Is it just gluttony? Is it that we all just woke up one day and decided, "You know, I think I'll start eating 400 more calories each day?" No! Obviously not. This increase in calorie consumption is biologically driven—it's because we *feel hungry and want to eat more*. And that simple fact—that this is an unconscious, biologically-driven process—changes everything! It changes the frame of fat gain from "we're eating too many calories so we just need to eat less" to "what are the environmental factors that drive our biology to over-consume calories, and how can we fix them?"

That is a massive shift in paradigm. It's the difference between trying to attain fat loss by fighting against your biology or by working with the intelligence of your body. And it's the difference between success and failure in your quest for lasting, sustainable fat loss.

If you say, "The problem is that we're eating too many calories, so we just need to eat less," your efforts at fat loss will be as futile as trying to clear away darkness with your hands. You will spend years spinning your wheels while torturing yourself through calorie deprivation, neurotic calorie counting, and hunger pangs, only to get nowhere except a cycle of losing and regaining the same 20 or 30 pounds.

Why? Because you've misunderstood the problem. The problem wasn't that we consciously decided to start eating more—it's that our biology drove us to do so! So the solution is not simply to consciously and forcibly eat less, it's to *eliminate the factors that caused us to start eating more in the first place!*

Yes, we are absolutely eating more calories now than we did a few decades ago, and yes, we are fatter. I'm not saying that calories don't matter. I'm simply suggesting that saying that "we're fat because we're eating more calories" is a lot like saying that "wind is caused by trees waving their branches." We must always avoid confusing the symptom with the cause. You can consciously starve your body of calories, but if the biological factors driving you to consume more calories are still present, they will eventually win out.

Fat gain is not just about calories—and those who claim that excess calories are the "cause" of fat gain, and that restricting calories is the solution, have missed the point entirely. **Something is driving us to unconsciously consume more calories, and that "something" is the real source of body fatness.**

And if we want to find a real, effective way of not only becoming lean but getting progressively leaner instead of just gaining the weight back, it's that something that you need to understand.

After all, we have the body fat set-point system that is supposed to be preventing us from getting fat, right?

How could we get fat if we have that body fat set-point system that I just explained to you?

Shouldn't this system prevent that?"

Well, you're right. The system *should* prevent that!

And that is precisely the problem. The system is broken. **Being overweight or obese is, by definition, a _dysfunctional_ body fat set-point system.**

People only get fat because something is either preventing the system from working or causing this system to malfunction.

This completely changes our paradigm of fat loss — this is the shift away from the Gluttony and Sloth theory of fat gain (i.e. "we're fat because we're lazy and have no self-control") to the Body Fat Set-Point Dysfunction theory of fat gain. This theory states that we're fat, not because we're simply overeating calories, but because of environmental factors that are driving our biology to overeat calories. Thus, the solution is clearly *not* just to fight our biology and forcibly restrict calories, but rather to remove the factors that are causing our biology to over-consume calories.

Before we get into the specific factors that cause the body fat set-point system to malfunction, we need to understand the *context* of this dysfunction more clearly. This leads me to three critical points:

- The table I showed you earlier depicting hunger and metabolism, and how the body responds to either a period of over-eating or under-eating, seems to imply that the body is *equally* good at defending against fat loss as it is fat gain. It isn't. The body fat set-point system, in general, is designed to defend against body fat *loss* much more than it is designed to prevent body fat gain. Unfortunately for you, if you're overweight, this system is *not* equally good at preventing fat loss and preventing fat gain. Our biology is wired in such a way that makes it somewhat easier to gain fat and far harder to lose it. This is not a mistake or coincidence. It makes a ton of sense if you consider the body fat set-point system in an evolutionary context. Not starving to death during a food shortage was more important to survival than not getting fat from overeating. The human genome is shaped by *survival demands*—that is, genes that help support survival to the environment get passed on and those that don't support survival get weeded out. This is why our body fat set-point system is better at defending against fat loss than it is at defending against fat gain. This means that the body fat set-point system is not likely to malfunction in its ability to prevent fat loss (it's exceptional at that), but it does have the potential to malfunction in terms of its ability to prevent fat gain—thus leaving us vulnerable to becoming overweight and obese.

- Our bodies are now *defending a higher set-point*. It's not just that we're eating more calories and we've gotten fatter, and therefore correcting the situation is just a matter of eating fewer calories. No, our bodies are now wired into higher set-point weights. This means we're fatter, and on top of just accumulating fat tissue, our body is now *resistant* to going back down to its previous leaner set-point. Even though it has an excess of body fat, it still perceives itself to be starving for energy, and fights against any attempt to get leaner. That is, it is defending its new higher set-point weight.

- The last thing we must consider in understanding why the body fat set-point system malfunctions is this: Bodyweight set-point malfunction is a *new* problem. Overweight and obesity have not become significant problems until the last 100 years, and really, only in the last 50 years have they become an epidemic. This immediately tells you that this is *not* some kind of genetic problem that makes us get fat automatically, regardless of our environment. As I explained before, wild animals and wild humans show us that the natural and default state of animals is effortless leanness without calorie counting or forced restriction. Universally, they have a near-zero incidence of overweight and obesity. This is critically important to understand: The *normal* and natural state of the body is to be lean, and when you are living in congruence with your genome, you stay *effortlessly* lean. The obesity epidemic is a completely new and unprecedented phenomenon unlike anything that has ever occurred in human history. Thus, something in the modern environment during the last 100 years is *obesogenic*, which means that something in our modern world is causing our bodyweight set-point systems to malfunction. As a result, our bodyweight set-points are being driven up.

Because the normal and natural state of the human body is to be effortlessly lean, there is one thing that's critical to realize here: The things that drive your body fat set-point up and cause overweight and obesity are things in the *modern environment*. So the solution to losing fat by driving the body fat set-point *down* is more about things that you *don't do*, rather than things that you *do* do.

What I mean is that people *will never* achieve lasting fat loss through *things you add on top of your normal routine*—like special fat-burning diet pills, fat-burning cardio and interval workouts, weight training, special fat-burning foods, supplements, 10-day green juice cleanses, or anything else that is about something *you do*.

It's not about goofy diet and exercise gimmicks that you add in for just "10 minutes a day" that magically transform your body while everything else about your lifestyle remains the same. It's not about some special diet trick, or "one weird trick," or so and so's magical "green superfood juice" concoction, or "5 weird foods" that get "rid of belly fat." That's why *all* of these fat-loss "solutions," which are based on getting you to do some positive action, are *failures* when it comes to long-term fat loss—because they do not remove the factors that are actually driving your body fat set-point up in the first place, and thus they just put you into a trap where you are fighting against your own biology. Fighting against your own biology is a fight you simply cannot win in the long-term.

Take all the fat-burning diet pills and appetite suppressants you want, do all the cardio and intervals you want, restrict calories all you want, do as many green juice fasts as you want, but as long as the obesogenic factors in the modern environment are still present in your life, they will eventually win out. You will lose weight for a period of time, and then you will slowly regain all the fat you lost—and probably some more on top of it.

All of the aforementioned strategies come out of the Gluttony and Sloth paradigm. And that paradigm, simply put, is wrong. All strategies that are built upon this foundation—the "eat fewer calories and burn more calories" paradigm—are destined for failure.

As Alan Watts stated at the beginning of this book (to paraphrase): "If you want to be successful solving a problem, you better be damn sure that you understand that problem completely. Because if you try to solve a problem you haven't fully understood, your efforts will be futile."

Remember, the *normal* state of humans is leanness, and the abnormal dysfunctional state of physiology is overweight and obesity. Thus, normalizing your physiology—driving the body fat set-point down—isn't about doing something on top of your current way of doing things, **it's first and foremost about _removing_ the factors in the modern environment that drive the body-fat set-point up.**

Thus, it's time to step out of the old, over-simplistic, worn-out and pseudoscientific paradigm of the Gluttony and Sloth theory of fat gain, and it's time to step into the future of fat loss: The Body Fat Set-Point Dysfunction theory of fat gain.

Let me show you what this really means in terms of how it differs from the other approaches to fat loss currently used by those in the fat loss industry.

Calories Do Matter. But You Should NOT Count Them! (A.K.A. How to Escape the Low-Calorie and Low-Carb Traps)

I have stated several times thus far in this book that deliberate calorie restriction is an extraordinarily ineffective and even counterproductive approach to fat loss. Yet, I've also stated that calories do indeed matter, and that in order to lose fat, you do need to be burning more calories than you take in.

To some, this may be confusing, as these statements may seem to be conflicting. How can it possibly be that calories matter—that to lose fat we need to be in a state where we are burning more calories than we're taking in—but that trying to do so by intentionally restricting calories below the body's needs virtually always results in failure?

The answer to that requires some clarification, so before we go into the practical aspects of my system, we first reconcile these seemingly-conflicting notions. Let me do that by showing you the two strategies that all other existing approaches to fat loss revolve around, and the traps inherent in those strategies—the low-calorie and low-carb diet traps.

Strategy #1: Tell people "you're fat because you're eating more calories than you burn" so the solution is to "eat fewer calories." (A.k.a. The Low Calorie Diet Trap)

I have already spent a large portion of this book explaining the low-calorie trap, so I'll keep this short.

The simple fact that you must eat fewer calories than you burn in order to lose fat from your body is true. However, when you analyze things at that very simplistic level like most people in the fitness and nutrition industries do, you are operating in an insidious trap where trying to do that will only cause short-term fat loss followed by metabolic slowdown and fat regain.

The only reason this approach is so popular is *not* because it actually works, but because most health, nutrition, and fitness authorities are painfully ignorant about the science of biological bodyweight regulation.

The Trap: Getting yourself into a never-ending battle against your own biology, suffering, with nothing to show for it all except an even slower metabolism than you started with, and an even fatter body.

Strategy # 2: Tell people "calories don't matter, and you can eat whatever you want if you use my magical diet." (A.k.a. The Low-Carb Diet Trap)

There is one more trap we should all be aware of: The Trap of "Calories don't matter if you use my special (insert various dieting gimmick here) diet."

No matter what anyone may tell you, the simple fact is that calories do matter if you want to lose weight. As the first law of thermodynamics clearly explains, matter/energy has to come from somewhere and it has to go somewhere. If you are eating more calories than you are burning, it is not possible for your body to somehow lose weight by some mystical process that defies basic thermodynamics.

Yet, there are many people out there trying to convince you of just that! There are lots of people out there trying to tell you that "calories don't matter" if you follow their special thermodynamics-transcending diet. The most popular of these diet gimmicks in recent years has been low-carb diets. We commonly hear low-carb gurus saying, "Calories don't matter as long as you don't eat those insulin-spiking carbs, because insulin is a fat-storing hormone. So if you don't eat carbs, then you can eat however much you want without getting fat!"

This is simply false. It has been proven wrong over and over again. If you eat 2,500 calories and you're only burning 2,000, it doesn't matter how few carbohydrates you eat, you're still going to get fat. As author of the *Fat Loss Bible*, Anthony Colpo, explains "Metabolic ward studies dating as far back as 1935 have repeatedly shown that when caloric intake is truly kept equal, there is absolutely no difference in fat-derived weight loss between low-carb and high-carb diets." [31] [32]

So how can we explain the weight loss that some people achieve on these fad diets? Basically, what's really going on here is this: They are simply telling you "calories don't matter" and then asking you to adhere to some diet rule that, as luck would have it, acts to *lower your total calorie intake*! In other words, they tell you it's not about calories and then basically trick you into lowering your calorie intake—e.g. "eat low-carb," "eat low-fat," "eat a vegan diet," "don't eat after 6pm," etc. There are a thousand different ways that diet book authors and other weight loss "experts" can use to get people to unknowingly lower their caloric intake without necessarily having to count or forcibly restrict calories.

Scientists have confirmed that when people go on typical low-carb diets, they end up eating significantly fewer calories overall.

---

31 Colpo, A. (2012, June 29). Finally, a study that proves a low-carb metabolic advantage? Yeah, Right... Retrieved from http://anthonycolpo.com/finally-a-study-that-proves-a-low-carb-metabolic-advantage-yeah-right/

32 Schoeller, D. A., & Buchholz, A. C. (2005). Energetics of obesity and weight control: Does diet composition matter? J Am Diet Assoc, 105(5 Suppl 1), S24-8.

Why? Simple: Most common low-carb diets (like nearly all "Paleo" diets) are high in protein and in whole foods, which are known factors that spontaneously drive overall calorie consumption down. Then, when these people lose weight, they think, "Wow, this low-carb thing is amazing. All you have to do is get rid of carbs and you'll get leaner!" Only, the same exact thing happens when someone eats a high-carb diet with ample protein and whole foods. The high protein and whole foods intake are responsible for this effect, not carbohydrate restriction. This has already been scientifically proven. The following study set out to control for the variability in protein intake that has tainted the results of many previous weight loss studies that low-carb gurus use to promote low-carb diets. This study asked a simple question: Is the weight loss people achieve on low-carb diets *actually* the result of carbohydrate restriction, or is it simply due to higher protein intake lowering overall calorie intake? Here's what they found:

BACKGROUND:

'Low-carb' diets have been suggested to be effective in body weight (BW) management. However, these diets are relatively high in protein as well.

OBJECTIVE:

To unravel whether body-weight loss and weight-maintenance depends on the high-protein or the 'low-carb' component of the diet...

CONCLUSION:

Body-weight loss and weight-maintenance depends on the high-protein, but not on the 'low-carb' component of the diet..."[33]

This was also the conclusion from the latest meta-analysis (comprehensive review of the scientific studies) on the subject just published in 2014: **"There is probably little or no difference in weight loss and changes in cardiovascular risk factors up to two years of follow-up when overweight and obese adults, with or without type 2 diabetes, are randomized to low CHO (low-carb) diets and Isoenergetic balance (higher carb diets that are equal in calories)."**[34]

In other words, a high-carbohydrate diet achieves the exact same weight loss effect when the same amount of protein and calories are eaten. There is nothing magical about carbohydrate restriction.

What is critical to understand is that any weight loss someone achieves on these fad diets has absolutely *nothing* to do with the magic of low-carb or the magic of low-fat or the magic of food combining or the magic of not eating after 6pm or the magic of Paleo or the magic of veganism. Nothing whatsoever! It is simply because all of these things end up causing people to lower their calorie intake without realizing it.

All of these approaches can work to cause fat loss. They work *to the extent* that someone actually does lower their calorie intake while eating this way. If someone does, these approaches *can*

---

33 Soenen, S., Bonomi, A. G., Lemmens, S. G., Scholte, J., Thijssen, M. A., van Berkum, F., & Westerterp-Plantenga, M. S. (2012). Relatively high-protein or 'low-carb' energy-restricted diets for body weight loss and body weight maintenance?. Physiol Behav. 107(3):374-80. doi: 10.1016/j.physbeh.2012.08.004.

34 Naude, C. Et al. (2014). Low Carbohydrate versus Isoenergetic Balanced Diets for Reducing Weight and Cardiovascular Risk: A Systematic Review and Meta-Analysis. Plos One. DOI: 10.1371/journal.pone.0100652

actually lead to sustainable fat loss, unlike the forced calorie restriction in #1.

However, misunderstanding the real factors underlying weight loss success is a treacherous mistake. When people started to figure out how to make low-carb jelly beans, low-carb ice cream, and low-carb pizza, and otherwise foolishly believing that it was the insulin/carbohydrates that were causing them to be fat rather than calories, being low-carb was not very helpful for fat loss. There are countless low-carbers (including some notable low-carb gurus) who are still overweight despite a decade of extreme "low-carb" eating. Why? Because they are eating the amount of calories they are burning. They are forcibly restricting carbohydrates (and feeling fatigued and suffering from low energy levels as a result of depriving themselves of carbohydrates) but failing to see any fat loss benefits from their carbohydrate deprivation.

The same thing happened in the 1990s when low-fat was all the rage. As soon as "low-fat" and "non-fat" processed foods hit the market and people started eating low-fat crackers and cookies to make up for the calories they were missing by restricting fat intake, low-fat diets stopped working for fat loss. In other words, when people think that eating low-carb or low-fat or vegan or whatever other diet fad provides some magical fat loss/health benefit that allows them to eat however much food they want while still remaining lean, their results come to a grinding halt. Then they don't understand why fat loss isn't occurring despite their strict low-carb (or other diet fad) eating.

Again, these little diet fads can work, but only to the extent that they cause you to sustainably eat fewer calories.

This situation where certain dietary changes can cause people to unconsciously lower their calorie intake isn't all bad, though. To be clear, I actually think higher protein intake and higher intake of whole foods are wonderful strategies to help you reach your fat loss goals. I am simply in favor of accurate scientific understanding of why things work the way they do and avoiding the perpetuation of carbohydrate-related confusion, ignorance, and pseudoscience. If you lost weight from eating a low-carb diet, it wasn't because the carbs you were eating were "making you fat," it was because you ate more *calories* than you do now.

The Trap: Failing to realize that the weight loss you achieved was due to eating fewer *calories*, and instead thinking it was because of the magic of low-carb (or low-fat, or vegan, or whatever else). In the long run, this ignorance can be disastrous and can result in years of fighting against your own cravings for carbohydrates, forcibly depriving your body of the nutrients it's crying out for, and ultimately getting nowhere when you could have easily gotten further without all that suffering, deprivation, fatigue, and fighting against your own biology. Or worse, if you start to eat beyond your caloric needs because you've been duped into thinking that calories no longer matter, if you're avoiding that "devil hormone" insulin, you can quickly find yourself getting fat again while being totally confused as to why it's happening (given all your strict avoidance of carbs) and maybe decide to restrict carbs *even more*.

Perhaps even more importantly, the trap here is really that these fad diets—low-carb in particular—can cause people to fail in the long run because they commonly result in hormonal problems and slow the metabolism, which predisposes one to future fat regain and health problems.

So if we want to avoid the low-calorie and low-carb diet traps, it's time for a new strategy...

Strategy #3: Identifying and eliminating the real causes of increased body fat set-point and enhancing cellular, hormonal, and metabolic function to actively drive down the body fat set-point without having to rely on calorie counting, forced deprivation, or fad diets.

This strategy is all about removing the factors that cause the body fat set-point system to malfunction in the first place. It's about enhancing cellular and metabolic health to send your biology the signal to effortlessly lower the body fat set-point.

This strategy allows you to avoid the trap of #2 (the low-carb and fad diet trap) by first realizing that the strategies in #2 only worked because they caused you to eat fewer calories, and second, by not screwing up your hormonal and metabolic function with low-carb, low-fat, and vegetarian dieting.

You are going to realize that calories *do* matter, and you're not going to make the mistake of thinking that once you adopt such and such (e.g. low-carb) diet that it will make you immune to calories, enabling you to magically eat an excess of calories without getting fat.

This strategy also allows you to avoid the trap of #1 (the low-calorie diet trap) because you won't actually be forcibly eating fewer calories. You won't have to count calories, and you won't have to suffer through hunger pangs. Thus, you will avoid the reason that strategy #1 fails in the long term—because of the metabolism slowdown that occurs with forced calorie restriction. Believe it or not, if you're going from a slow metabolism and a sedentary lifestyle to what I recommend here, you may even achieve fat loss (i.e. be in a state where you're burning more calories than you're taking in) while eating *more calories* than you're currently eating.

By using this strategy, you actually have a real, genuine, sustainable fat loss plan that is proven to not only cause fat loss, but to keep it off in the long term.

This is really the *only* way of modifying your nutrition that leads to sustainable and lasting fat loss while improving your health and speeding up your metabolism rather than slowing it down. No suffering, no fighting against your own cravings and hunger pangs, and no forced deprivation necessary.

If you want lasting, sustainable, and effortless fat loss (and optimal health), then you want strategy #3.

One important thing to realize is that this approach typically *does not work as fast* as calorie counting and forced starvation. If you starve your body of calories, you can achieve massive weight loss of 20 or 30 pounds in a month or two. So that method does have great appeal to the magic-pill mentality (which is unfortunately all too common), and that's why so many millions are continuously being duped into using that method while being unaware that they are eventually destined to regain back all the weight they lost.

This isn't the fastest way to get lean (starvation is the fastest way to get lean), but this is the *right* way to go about losing fat if you expect it to be permanent.

So, instead of telling you to do something that will get great short-term results and terrible long-term results, I am proposing the right way to lose fat—the way that gets you real, lasting fat loss success. This is a *real* fat loss solution.

Want out of the low-calorie and low-carb diet traps? Well, then it's all about enhancing cellular health, re-engaging the body fat set-point system, and sending your biology the signal to lower your body fat set-point!

The True Path to Lasting Fat Loss is Not Starvation - It's Lowering the Body Fat Set-Point!

Shifting out of the Gluttony and Sloth paradigm of fat gain into the Body Fat Set-Point Dysfunction paradigm of fat gain creates a big shift in how we attempt to solve the issue of fat loss. What is that shift? Simply put: Fat loss is no longer about trying to fight against your biology by starving it of calories—it's about lowering the body's preferred body fat set-point. And this is quite different than starving the body of calories.

If the cause of fat gain were simply calories—that we are consciously eating too many of them— then the answer really would be as simple as just making the decision to eat less of them. But it's not that simple. The problem is that it is a **biologically driven** overconsumption of calories. While calories *do* matter— that is, we are fatter because we are consuming more calories today than we did 50 years ago—the problem is *not simply* "too many calories." Thus, the real question is this: Why are we over-consuming calories?

Guyenet explains:

> **"Because the system that should be defending a low fat mass is now defending a high fat mass. Therefore, the solution is not simply to restrict calories, or burn more**

calories through exercise, but to try to "reset" the system that decides what fat mass to defend. Restricting calories isn't necessarily a good solution because the body will attempt to defend its set-point, whether high or low, by increasing hunger and decreasing its metabolic rate. That's why low-calorie diets, and most diets in general, typically fail in the long term. It's miserable to fight hunger every day." [35]

What should be abundantly clear at this point is that the "burn more calories than you take in" approach to fat loss is not an intelligent or effective approach to fat loss. It attempts to get fat loss by entering into a fight against the body fat set-point system—by fighting against your biology and trying to starve it.

As Guyenet goes on to explain:

"Therefore, what we need for sustainable fat loss is not starvation; we need a treatment that lowers the fat mass set-point. There are several criteria that this treatment will have to meet to qualify:

1. It must cause fat loss
2. It must not involve *deliberate* calorie restriction
3. It must maintain fat loss over a long period of time
4. It must not be harmful to overall health." [36]

What he has outlined here are the fundamental principles for long-term fat loss success—these four principles are the blueprint to a new scientific approach to lasting fat loss. Elaborating further on those points, what we need is something that:

1. Actually works to cause fat loss (because if it doesn't do this, all the other factors become largely meaningless).

---

35 Guyenet, S. (2010, January 31). The body fat setpoint, part iv: Changing the setpoint. Retrieved from
http://wholehealthsource.blogspot.com/2010/01/body-fat-setpoint-part-iv-changing.html

36 Guyenet, S. (2010, January 31). The body fat setpoint, part iv: Changing the setpoint. Retrieved from
http://wholehealthsource.blogspot.com/2010/01/body-fat-setpoint-part-iv-changing.html

2. Causes fat loss, but *not* by forcibly depriving yourself of food when you're hungry. Instead, it causes fat loss by effortlessly and non-forcibly driving the body to be in a state where it is burning more fat than it is storing.
3. Needs to be a *habit* that you can sustain on an ongoing basis for the rest of your life— not just a temporary weight-loss diet that relies on willpower and deprivation of various kinds.
4. Actually enhances your cellular health rather than something that damages it.
5. And I would also add a 5th requirement (based on my own research and experimentation in this area): It must *not* result in metabolic slowdown—and ideally should result in a *faster* metabolism.

I want to point out something before I go any further: All the diet and weight loss plans out there currently fail in at least one of these five principles. Most weight loss diets out there do work to cause fat loss (in the short-term), so they technically succeed in Guyenet's first principle. (Note: Achieving short-term fat loss is really quite easy—all you have to do is starve yourself. The problem is that the fat doesn't *stay off.*) But virtually all of them fail in at least one of the other four principles—and typically they fail in *all four!*

Most of the weight-loss gurus promote deliberate calorie deprivation of some kind—either calorie counting, conscious portion control, or restriction on the number of meals you eat each day—and all of these ways to consciously lower calorie intake have an abysmal failure rate. This means they fail principle #2. They fail principle #3 because they typically rely upon forced calorie deprivation and suffering through hunger, and they are often nutrient-deficient diets (e.g. low-carb diets, low-fat diets, simultaneous low-carb and low-fat diets, etc.), so they require you to fight against your cravings for the nutrient you are restricting, and thus, they are not sustainable. The simple fact that there are typically health side effects that result from long-term low-fat, vegan, and low-carb dieting means that they fail principle #4. And all of them fail miserably when it comes to #5, because they almost always result in metabolic slowdown due to the forced calorie restriction or restriction of macronutrients (carbohydrates in particular). Thus, they end up causing fat regain.

So is there anything that actually meets the criteria outlined above as the essential criteria for weight loss success?

Well, after years of research and experimentation (with myself and my clients), I have developed what I believe is the only system in existence that succeeds in all five of these principles— a system that doesn't just starve the body into fat loss, but **actually lowers the body fat set-point**!

The real path to lasting fat loss success is not fighting against your biology, it's working with it. It is simply re-engaging the body fat set-point system by removing the factors that caused it to dysfunction in the first place!

And it does this:

- Without being damaging to health (like most weight loss diets), but actually enhancing it dramatically.
- Without relying on forced calorie restriction and suffering through hunger. (No fighting through cravings and suffering through hunger pangs necessary!)
- Without macronutrient restriction (i.e. low-fat or low-carb diets).
- Without causing metabolic slowdown and fat regain, but actually speeding up the metabolism!

With that said, let's now get into the specific factors that cause our body fat set-point system to dysfunction. In order to eliminate them, we must first figure out what they are.

Identifying and Removing the Causes of Fat Gain

So now that we understand that lasting fat loss is all about re-engaging the body fat set-point by removing the factors from the modern environment that cause it to dysfunction, here's what we need to do:

1. Identify those factors in the modern environment that are causing your bodyweight set-point to increase.
2. *Remove* those factors from your environment. What happens next is that your body fat set-point system re-engages, and it drives your body fat set-point down *effortlessly*. Removing these factors causes fat loss without any forced calorie restriction or suffering through hunger, and without all the negative metabolic adaptations that come with dieting (fatigue, loss of muscle mass, and decreased NEAT/metabolism).

Before we get into the specific lifestyle factors that drive fat gain, I would like to address an important issue: Genetics.

There has been much talk in recent years of the search to discover the "fat gene(s)"—the specific genes that "cause" us to become fat. Of course, genetics play an enormous role in just about everything related to human health, including obesity. *All* human diseases can be said to have a "genetic component." However, outside of true genetic diseases (i.e. Down's syndrome, Klinefelter's syndrome, etc) what genetics determine (to either a small or relatively large degree) is your **susceptibility** to a given disease. *Susceptibility* to becoming obese is of course, largely genetically determined, but common obesity and fat gain is most definitely *not* a "genetic condition." We can see this rather clearly by a few facts:

1. Obesity epidemics do not exist in populations still living a traditional lifestyle.
2. When those same populations are introduced to the modern Western lifestyle and diet, they all of the sudden begin to become obese and diabetic. (This has been seen in countless modernizing societies all over the world over the last century).
3. The simple fact that in the U.S., obesity rates have quadrupled in half a century—a blink of an eye in evolutionary time. Genetics have not changed during that time span, but we have seen a radical shift in our *environment* (i.e. lifestyle) unlike anything that has ever occurred in human history. When there is an abrupt shift in just a few generations where all of the sudden huge amounts of people become fat and obese, and there has been no concurrent shift in genetics, it's telling us that other factors (i.e. not genetics) are causing the increase.

To put it simply, obesity is a modern epidemic that is triggered primarily by environmental factors. In an obesity-inducing environment (e.g. the modern Western world), some individuals will, of course, be genetically more prone to actually become more overweight/obese than other individuals. This, however, does not mean that obesity "is hereditary." It means simply that if you insert a large group of people into an environment that is obesogenic, certain individuals will get more fat than others—a few might not become very fat at all, and a few might become extremely fat. The key point though, is that if you take that same group and put them in an environment where they are living close to how most traditional hunter-gatherer human populations live, essentially *none* of those people—not even the individuals who are the *most genetically prone to obesity*—will become obese. The environmental triggers for fat gain are still needed to become fat. People aren't becoming fat because they're genetically programmed to become fat. Genes are not destiny when it comes to how fat or lean you are. Environmental conditions are the key player here. To put all this simply, the equation is this:

Modern Lifestyle + Genetic susceptibility = Fat Gain

On a practical level, for those actually seeking to lose fat, I do not find the focus on the hereditary factors in obesity to be particularly useful. In fact, I find it to be a largely misleading and disempowering viewpoint that generally just distracts from what is the much more important factor: Lifestyle.

It is a fact that we all must simply accept that some of us are more genetically susceptible to fat gain and will tend to put on fat when others with the same habits may not. How do you know if you're genetically susceptible? Well, if you're overweight, more than likely you have at least some degree of genetic susceptibility to fat gain. That's just something we all have to accept, since we can't do anything about it.

The critical thing to take away from this understanding is that while we cannot do anything to change our genetic proneness to fat gain, we *can* do a whole lot to address the lifestyle factors that impact the expression of our genes, and we can make sure that our "fat genes" are switched off.

So your choice is really simple: You can wait around for technology to advance to the point where scientists are able to change our genetics to dictate how fat or lean we are regardless of how we eat, move, and live our lives. (Unlimited pizza and cheesecake while having six-pack abs is something I would love to have too!). Or, perhaps more intelligently, you can address the factors you do have control over—your lifestyle.

Now that we accurately understand the place of genetics, let's start with identifying precisely what those factors are. The factors that cause the body fat set-point system to malfunction can be divided into two general categories: Neurological and

Cellular/Hormonal. By "Neurological Causes," I mean things that are happening primarily in the brain. And by "Cellular/Hormonal," I mean things that are happening primarily in the cells and bloodstream.

First, let's look at the neurological causes.

The Neurological Causes of Fat Gain

So what are these things going on in the brain that drive the body fat set-point up? There are several neurological causes of obesity:

1. High Food Reward
2. High Food Variety
3. Circadian Rhythm Disruption

1. HIGH FOOD REWARD

What is "food reward?" Well, it's pretty simple actually: It's food that tastes really good. Like, really, *really* good.

When you taste something that makes you say, "Oh my god, that is frickin' delicious," that's highly rewarding food. Why is it called "highly rewarding" food? Because it makes the *reward center* of your brain light up! When the reward center of your brain lights up, dopamine is released, and you feel the sensation of pleasure.

Now, pleasure is not all bad. In fact, it's rather good and important for you to feel it often. However, our brain is wired for a certain threshold of rewarding stimuli, and certain kinds of things stimulate the reward center of our brain in an unnaturally intense way, which can cause problems.

What kind of things?

Addictive drugs work by creating this excessively intense stimulation of the reward center of the brain. Highly rewarding processed foods also do it.

When you stimulate the brain in this way with highly rewarding food, it can drive addiction in much the same way that addictive drugs do, thus resulting in you wanting more and more of that thing. [37] [38] [39] [40]

When it comes to drugs, the end result is drug addiction and the whole set of consequences that go along with that. When it comes to highly rewarding, addictive food, the end result is essentially obesity (and its associated complications, like type II diabetes).

To put it simply: A high food reward diet drives chronic overconsumption of calories, and thus, leads to fat gain. [41]

What I'm talking about here is food addiction. I do not mean this in the hyperbolic way we typically use the word "addiction" in conversation—like, "I'm addicted to these Cheetos 'cause they're so good." I mean addiction in a very literal, scientific sense. In exactly the same way that it's possible to get addicted to cocaine or heroin, it's possible to get addicted to food. Yes, really. It's not true chemical dependence, but the neurological changes

---

37 Johnson PM, Kenny PJ. Dopamine D2 receptors in addiction-like reward dysfunction and compulsive eating in obese rats. Nat Neurosci. 2010 Mar 28. [Epub ahead of print]

38 Scripps Research Institute (2010, March 29). Compulsive eating shares addictive biochemical mechanism with cocaine, heroin abuse, study shows. ScienceDaily. Retrieved April 16, 2010, from http://www.sciencedaily.com/releases/2010/03/100328170243.htm

39 Daniells, S. (2010, March 29). Food addiction: Fat may rewire brain like hard drugs. Retrieved from http://www.foodnavigator.com/Science-Nutrition/Food-addiction-Fat-may-rewire-brain-like-hard-drugs/?c=DFrDdGqlXj9PxLeDW0x8cw%3D%3D&utm_source=newsletter_daily&utm_medium=email&utm_campaign=Newsletter%2BDaily

40 Pearson, A. (2010, March 28). Junk-fed rats have 'drug addict' brains. Retrieved from http://www.newscientist.com/article/dn18706-junkfed-rats-have-drug-addict-brains.html?DCMP=OTC-rss&nsref=health#.U2fv44GSzHk.

41 Guyenet, S. (2011, October 1). The case for the food reward hypothesis of obesity, part I. Retrieved from http://wholehealthsource.blogspot.com/2011/10/case-for-food-reward-hypothesis-of.html .

in the brain are extremely similar, as are the end behaviors. The same thing that happens with cocaine or nicotine can also happen with food—your brain can become wired into neurological addiction. But this doesn't happen with just any food—only with what obesity researchers call "highly-rewarding" foods.

So what's going on with processed "highly rewarding" foods and our brain?

When you do things that give you pleasure—like cocaine or heroin, for example—you are lighting up the hedonic (i.e. hedonistic, or pleasure) part of the brain in an unnaturally intense way. Do this with a decent frequency, and soon enough you'll find yourself craving that feeling again. And, moreover, the reward threshold (the amount of that substance you need to feel a certain amount of pleasure) goes up, so you end up needing more of the same thing to feel that same amount of pleasure.[42] That's the beginning of a vicious cycle similar to what happens in drug addiction. You may not have a true physiological chemical dependence as in drug addiction, but the end behaviors--craving and seeking out more and more of that substance--are essentially the same. You give into the craving again and again until you are enslaved by your own brain, and the pleasure center in your brain is running the show and making decisions as far as what to eat and when.

Why does this cause the body fat set-point system to dysfunction?

Well, it's not so much that it causes the body fat set-point system to "dysfunction"—it's really more that it just overrides it altogether. Think of it this way: Your body fat set-point system works through just a few simple mechanisms--hunger/fullness, and increasing/decreasing the metabolism. Just through modifying hunger and metabolism, the body can constantly ensure that calories in equal calories out, and bodyweight stays stable. When your body is low on nutrients, you feel hungry and

---

42 Kenny, P. (2011). Reward Mechanisms in Obesity: New Insights and Future Directions. Neuron. 69(4):664-679.

eat more. When you're full with nutrients, you eat less. It's constantly modifying your eating behavior *according to your body's biological need*. That last part is crucial to understand. Now, let's think about how neurological addiction might change this natural regulation of eating behaviors in accordance with biological need. When you eat highly rewarding processed food regularly, you start eating in order to give yourself neurological pleasure, rather than because your body requires fuel. This causes you to lose touch with the signals from your body fat set-point system. It causes your eating behaviors to become *progressively dissociated from eating according to your body's biological need*. As a result of eating to give yourself neurological pleasure, you become numb to the signals telling you to stop eating, and instead start listening to your brain's cravings for more pleasure, which leads you to eat beyond your body's biological need. Essentially, what's going on is that the hedonic system in your brain is overriding the body fat set-point feedback system.

What are the most highly-rewarding foods? Generally speaking, modern processed foods are the most rewarding—typically in a combination of refined sugars and fats, mixed with artificial flavorings that are professionally engineered to maximize the reward factor in the brain. These are the foods that have the potential to be *hyper-rewarding* to the extent that they can actually start altering our brain's function around eating behaviors and change how much total food we eat on a daily basis. Sugar by itself is not especially rewarding, though it is moderately so. Fat by itself is not especially rewarding, though it is moderately so. And artificial flavorings aren't especially rewarding by themselves, either. But combine fats and sugars in a refined form (stripped of natural fibers for example), and lace the combination with a bunch of artificial flavorings that are professionally engineered with the specific intent to maximize food reward, and well, you have some extraordinarily rewarding food.

Just to give you a small sample of what I'm talking about here, let's take a look at a common list of ingredients for a strawberry milkshake at a fast food restaurant:

"Milk Fat, Milk Non-Fat, Sugar, Whey Sweet, Corn Syrup High Fructose, Corn Syrup, Flavor(s) Natural and Artificial Vanilla, Guar Gum, Mono and Diglycerides, Cellulose Gum, Sodium Phosphate, Carrageenan, Strawberry(ies) Syrup, Corn Syrup, Water, Corn Syrup High Fructose, Citric Acid, Artificial Flavor, Sodium Benzoate Preservative, Red 40"

Okay, pretty bad, huh? But maybe not absolutely terrible—it could be worse, right?

Let's take a closer look at just *one* of those ingredients— "artificial flavor." I wonder what's in that. Here's the list of ingredients in that specific "artificial flavor" used in this restaurant's milkshake:

amyl acetate, amyl butyrate, amyl valerate, anethol, anisyl formate, benzyl acetate, benzyl isobutyrate, butyric acid, cinnamyl isobutyrate, cinnamyl valerate, cognac essential oil, diacetyl, dipropyl ketone, ethyl butyrate, ethyl cinnamate, ethyl heptanoate, ethyl heptylate, ethyl lactate, ethyl methylphenylglycidate, ethyl nitrate, ethyl propionate, ethyl valerate, heliotropin, hydroxyphrenyl- 2-butanone (10% solution in alcohol), ionone, isobutyl anthranilate, isobutyl butyrate, lemon essential oil, maltol, 4-methylacetophenone, methyl anthranilate, methyl benzoate, methyl cinnamate, methyl heptine carbonate, methyl naphthyl ketone, methyl salicylate, mint essential oil, neroli essential oil, nerolin, neryl isobutyrate, orris butter, phenethyl alcohol, rose, rum ether, undecalactone, vanillin and solvent.

It is a chemical cocktail of over 50 ingredients mixed in precise amounts and professionally engineered to maximize the amount of fireworks in the reward center of your brain.

A hundred years ago, a strawberry milkshake would've consisted of milk and strawberries. Today, it's a mix of dozens of chemicals professionally engineered by scientists in a lab to make sure it is incredibly tasty and hyperrewarding. The more rewarding it is, the more it will drive the consumer to eat more of it (well beyond what their body actually needs), and the more that business has a repeat customer. So it's important to recognize that it's actually in the interest of every producer of processed food products to produce the most rewarding food possible. In fact, that's an understatement. Because we live in a capitalistic society, there is actually a Darwinian survival-of-the-fittest type of evolutionary process going on in the food industry. **It is *only* those products which have the strongest neurological reward effects that survive on the market place--the less rewarding products will slowly fade out of existence.** Moreover, the most highly rewarding and calorie-dense foods also happen to be cheapest--and the amount of calories than one can purchase per dollar is far higher now than it was just 30 or 40 years ago. Thus the very economics of our society drive a progressively more obesogenic environment.

In fact, one interesting scientific literature review suggests that more so than any other factor, fat gain is the result of food choices dictated by economics. It's called "The Real Contribution of Added Sugars and Fats to Obesity."

To pull out a few highlights from the abstract:

"Obesity rates in the United States are a function of socioeconomic status. Higher rates are found among groups with lower educational and income levels, among racial and ethnic minorities, and in high-poverty areas. Yet, the relation between obesity, nutrition, and diet continues to be viewed in biologic terms, with the search for likely causes focused on consumption of specific macronutrients, foods, or food groups…Plausible physiologic mechanisms have included the metabolic effects of dietary components, mostly sugars and fats, on regulation of food intake and deposition of body fat. **However, the evidence could not have been convincing since the blame for rising obesity rates seems to shift regularly, every 10 years or so, from fats to sugars and then back again. … This review demonstrates that much of past epidemiologic research is consistent with a single parsimonious explanation: obesity has been linked repeatedly to consumption of low-cost foods.** Refined grains, added sugars, and added fats are inexpensive, good tasting, and convenient. In other words, **the low cost of dietary energy (dollars/megajoule), rather than specific food, beverage, or macronutrient choices, may be the main predictor of population weight gain.**"[43]

While food costs are undoubtedly partially at play, the bigger factor at play here is that low-cost processed foods are typically highly rewarding and thus drive up overall calorie consumption tremendously (while also disrupting the brain's ability to regulate energy balance).[44] [45] [46]

An important note: This effect has nothing to do with carbohydrates, grains, sugars, or insulin—as many low-carb gurus like to promulgate. Foods rich in carbohydrates and natural sugars do have moderate reward value, but fatty foods like cheese, bacon, and peanut butter can be just as rewarding as sugary foods. Refined industrial food products that are professionally engineered to maximize palatability and reward are the big players here—not "carbs" or "sugars" or "fats." Strip some foods of their natural fiber content, condense the calories with a mixture of refined fats and sugars, add in some artificial chemical mixtures to ramp up the taste factor, and the pleasure center of the brain is gonna light up like a Christmas tree. Do that often, and you will have a hard time getting enough of the stuff!

Remember, I told you that it is specifically factors in the *modern* world that are driving obesity. Processed food is probably the most significant culprit behind the obesity epidemic. Processed, "highly-rewarding" food is a major factor that overrides how your body fat set-point system acts to drive your body fat set-point up. This has been made abundantly clear all over the world—as soon as a traditional tribal society is introduced to processed foods, they see rates of overweight and obesity go

---

43 http://www.ncbi.nlm.nih.gov/pubmed/17591599
44
http://www.foodandnutritionresearch.net/index.php/fnr/article/view/5144/5755
45 http://www.sciencedirect.com/science/article/pii/S0031938404001842
46 http://jn.nutrition.org/content/133/3/831S.full

from basically nonexistent to skyrocketing all the way up to levels in the U.S. In the U.S. itself, processed food and fast food consumption has paralleled the obesity epidemic perfectly—as we eat more refined and processed commercially prepared foods, we consume more calories, and as we consume more calories, we get fatter. This trend has been witnessed over and over again throughout the world.[47] [48]

As obesity scientist Rudolph Leibel and other researchers involved in the landmark study "Obesity and Leptin Resistance: Distinguishing Cause from Effect" explain: **"During the last 50 years, two major changes have shifted the energy balance equation: the decreased requirement for physical energy expenditure and the increased availability and abundance of palatable calorically-dense foods.** A common research model of obesity investigators, diet-induced obesity (DIO), mirrors the ubiquity of highly palatable calorie-dense foods in modern societies. In this paradigm, animals remain lean when maintained on standard chow, but increase their caloric intake and rapidly gain adipose mass when provided a calorically dense diet (generally high in both fat and sugar content). While genetic predispositions to DIO clearly exist (some rodent strains gain little weight on high-calorie compared to normal chow, while others rapidly progress to obesity) (51), **it is the availability of a highly palatable diet that drives overeating and subsequent obesity in these models."**[49]

The reason for it is simple: Processed food progressively dissociates your eating behaviors from your biological need for

47 Guyenet, S. (2008, May 15). Lessons from the Pima Indians. Retrieved from http://wholehealthsource.blogspot.com/2008/05/lessons-from-pima-indians.html.

48 Guyenet, S. (2009, January 19). The Tokelau Island Migrant Study: Diabetes. Retrieved from http://wholehealthsource.blogspot.com/2009/01/tokelau-island-migrant-study-diabetes.html.

49 http://www.ncbi.nlm.nih.gov/pmc/articles/PMC2967652/

fuel—it causes you to consume food to give your brain pleasure, not because your cells actually need fuel. This is a major factor driving chronic overconsumption of calories and fat gain.

Everyone has heard from the weight loss gurus at some point some vague notion like "Don't eat processed junk food—it's bad for you." Well, it's true, but now you actually understand *why*. In my 15 years of studying this field, I've literally never heard anyone intelligently explain why 500 calories of processed food is different from 500 calories of fruits and vegetables. The reason that the same amount of calories from processed food is different from whole food is because the processed food is affecting you differently on a neurological level. Highly rewarding processed food overstimulates the hedonic area in your brain so strongly that it is affecting your physiology completely differently. And, over time, it overrides the body fat set-point system and causes you to become out of harmony with eating according to your body's actual biological need. The result for those of us who become neurologically wired to eat more and more rewarding processed foods is simple: We get fat.

2. HIGH FOOD VARIETY

There is a second neurological factor aside from highly rewarding foods that is driving the obesity epidemic on a neurological level: food variety.

Have you ever been full after eating dinner, having absolutely stuffed yourself, and then suddenly found room for more when offered dessert? Have you ever been to an all-you-can-eat buffet and noticed the "unbuckle-your-pants syndrome," where people can gorge themselves on a huge amount of different foods? Well, these are both due to something called "food-specific fullness." That simply means that we feel "full," but only for specific foods. We may feel full on dinner, for example, but not feel full for dessert.

So, as if just having highly processed foods that are professionally engineered to maximize neurological reward weren't enough, in the modern world, we have a combination of hyper-rewarding foods *and* an endless *variety* of those hyper-rewarding foods. What is the result?

One recent study gives us a clue:

The study[50] is titled "Variety in the Diet Enhances Intake in a Meal and Contributes to the Development of Obesity in the Rat." Dr. Barbara Rolls and colleagues examined the effect of both rewarding foods and food variety on food intake and fat gain in rats. They tested six different diets:

1. Regular rat chow
2. Rat chow plus crackers
3. Rat chow plus cookies
4. Rat chow plus chocolate
5. Rat chow plus crackers, cookies, or chocolate, with each of the palatable foods given in succession (i.e. chow plus crackers, then chow plus cookies, etc.).
6. Rat chow plus crackers, cookies, and chocolate all at the same time.

As we might expect, adding a very rewarding food to the diet (crackers, cookies, or chocolate, in this case) increased food intake. Now, here's the kicker: Adding *multiple* rewarding foods together increased food intake significantly beyond just one of the rewarding foods. So we can see that both variety and food reward contribute to food intake.

After seven weeks, the rats eating the high food reward and high food variety diet gained close to triple the amount of weight of rats eating regular rat chow, and significantly more weight than rats eating just one rewarding food.

Numerous studies, including human studies, have shown the same result:

"Increased variety in the food supply may contribute to the development and maintenance of obesity. Thirty-nine studies examining dietary variety, energy intake, and body composition

---

50 Rolls, B. J., Van Duijvenvoorde, P. M., & Rowe, E. A. (1983). Variety in the diet enhances intake in a meal and contributes to the development of obesity in the rat. Physiol Behav. 31(1), 21-7.

are reviewed. Animal and human studies show that food consumption increases when there is more variety in a meal or diet and that greater dietary variety is associated with increased body weight and fat."[51]

People in tribal societies eating their traditional diets eat simple whole-food meals with just a few foods at the most, not three- or four-course meals with lots of different foods to try. They didn't have grocery stores around every corner with an endless variety of foods—they had a very small range of foods that they typically ate day in and day out. I went trekking in the Himalayas recently, and I can tell you from staying with the Sherpa people in the mountain villages that probably more than 90% of their diet is a meal called *daal bat*, which is basically rice and lentils (sometimes with a carrot and potato curry). Over and over again, it's the same exact rice and lentil meal, meal after meal, every day, year after year. Like I said, traditional populations eat *simple* diets and *simple* meals.

The introduction of different appetizers, entrees, desserts, and endless options of variety each day (especially endless variety of highly processed rewarding foods) is not congruent with our food-specific fullness system and drives us to *eat beyond our body's biological need*. In other words, it's a factor that prevents our body fat set-point system from working properly, and over time drives our body fat set-points up.

The last thing that's important to mention here is this: There are many obesity researchers who now believe that even without exploring any other causes of fat gain, high food reward and high food variety can explain the entire obesity epidemic by themselves. In other words, even if you never got into any other aspect of the physiology or hormonal aspects of obesity, and you *only* knew about highly-rewarding foods and high food variety, this knowledge alone is quite possibly enough to bring a total halt

---

51 Raynor, H. A., & Epstein, L. H. (2001). Dietary variety, energy regulation, and obesity. Psychol Bull. 127(3), 325-41.

to the obesity epidemic. That's how important and powerful eating a simple diet of whole unprocessed foods is.

3. DISRUPTED CIRCADIAN RHYTHM

There is one more neurological factor responsible for driving up the body fat set-point: poor sleep and disrupted circadian rhythm.

Why is this a neurological factor? Well, circadian rhythm is largely regulated by the brain (in particular, the "clock" that regulates our 24 hour sleep/wake cycle is in the suprachiasmatic nucleus in the hypothalamus). It's not critical that you remember the name of this specific part of the brain, but what is important is that you understand that circadian rhythm is regulated by the brain in response to environmental cues that tell it when it's daytime and when it's nighttime.

Several studies have now linked poor sleep and disrupted circadian rhythm with fat gain.[52][53][54] Sleep is a huge factor, and if you don't sleep well, you're going to have trouble losing fat no matter how good your diet and exercise are. In Wiley and Formby's book *Lights Out: Sleep, Sugar, and Survival*, they make the case that disrupted circadian rhythm is a major contributor to most modern day degenerative diseases like obesity, diabetes, heart disease, and cancer—just as big of a contributor as what we eat and how we exercise.

But you might be wondering how sleep relates to fat gain, since fat gain must be driven by an overconsumption of calories relative to how many are being burned—thus, sleep would have to affect the calories in-calories out equation in some way.

---

52 Cappuccio, F. P., Taggart, F. M., Kandala, N., Currie, A., Peile, E., Stranges, S., & Miller, M. A. (2008). Meta-analysis of short sleep duration and obesity in children and adults. Sleep. 31(5), 619–626.

53 Knutson, K. L. (2012). Does inadequate sleep play a role in vulnerability to obesity? Am J Hum Biol. 24(3), 361-71. doi: 10.1002/ajhb.22219.

54 Buxton, O. M., Cain, S. W., O'Connor, S. P., Porter, J. H., Duffy, J. F., Wang, W. ... Shea, S. A. (2012). Adverse metabolic consequences in humans of prolonged sleep restriction combined with circadian disruption. Sci. Transl. Med. 4, 129ra43.

It turns out that poor sleep actually affects *both*. It tends to de-regulate appetite and drive excess consumption of calories (particularly from highly rewarding foods),[55] and it tends to cause fatigue (and perhaps metabolism slowdown), which decreases calories burned. Together, this creates a powerful physiological tendency towards fat storage.

So what causes disrupted circadian rhythm?

Our modern world just so happens to be built perfectly for throwing off the physiological systems that regulate our circadian rhythm.

The major factor that disrupts the circadian rhythm is abnormal light rhythms. It is also the single most important factor you need to correct if you want to restore normal circadian rhythm. Organisms evolved to adjust themselves to the rise and fall of the sun in a physiological cycle known as the circadian rhythm ("circadian" means "about a day"). Once artificial light started altering the length of a daylight cycle, our rise and fall became somewhat dissociated from the rise and fall of the sun, and the average night's sleep decreased from around nine consistent hours to roughly seven, often varying from one night to the next. This state of affairs is the primary culprit for why so many people in modern society struggle with insomnia. While electricity and efficient lighting have clearly provided major benefits to society, these benefits come with a price: the betrayal of your inner clock.

To be more specific, when it comes to light exposure, there are basically two light problems that disrupt circadian rhythm:

1. Deficiency in sunlight exposure during daylight hours. We need sunlight for numerous reasons, like making vitamin D (from the sun's UV rays), stimulation of cellular energy production (largely from light in the red wavelengths), and melatonin suppression (from light in the blue wavelengths).

---

55 Guyenet, S. (2013, October 9). Sleep and genetic obesity risk. Retrieved from http://wholehealthsource.blogspot.com/2013/10/sleep-and-genetic-obesity-risk.html

Sunlight is bioactive! It affects numerous aspects of our physiology and is an essential requirement for health. The deficiency of red and UV wavelengths can result in deficient cellular energy production and the problems associated with low vitamin D, but as sleep and circadian rhythm are concerned, the big problem is blue light. Blue light is what the circadian clock is wired to respond to. Why? Because the only time an organism was exposed to light in the blue wavelengths (prior to the invention of electricity), was from the sun—particularly around midday. You know, like bright sun and the blue sky. If blue light photons were entering the eyeballs and feeding back into the brain, that meant that the sun was up and it was time to be awake. So what happens when you spend all day indoors (as many of us in the modern world do)? Well, we do not get enough of the stimulus that tells our brains "this is daytime, the time to be awake," and melatonin (the hormone that should be suppressed during daylight hours) is not adequately suppressed. End result: Circadian Rhythm is disrupted.

2. Too much blue light after the sun goes down. The problem isn't just as simple as spending too much time indoors, however. We now have artificial light sources, like TVs, cell phones, and computer screens, emitting light in the blue light spectrum long after the sun goes down—which enters our eyes and feeds back into the brain where it tells the brain "it's daytime," and as a result, melatonin is suppressed. This is a good thing during the middle of the day, but a pretty terrible thing when we have lots of blue light entering our eyes after sunset. Normally, when darkness arrives after the sun goes down, melatonin goes up, and we get tired and ready for sleep, as our ancestors had done for hundreds of thousands of years prior to the invention of electricity. Due to modern artificial light sources, we now have blue light pouring into our eyes for hours after sunset.

The end result: Our circadian clock doesn't get an adequate signal of what is day and what is night, and we end up fatigued when we shouldn't be (during the day) and too awake when we shouldn't be (at night). Over time, this damages our health, and creates subtle changes in the calories in-calories out equation that drive fat gain and hinder fat loss.

While light is the primary factor that throws off our circadian clock, there are some other causes as well, such as lack of movement (which I explore in the Movement Deficiency sections of this book) and micronutrient deficiencies. The primary micronutrient deficiency that contributes to faulty circadian rhythm is magnesium.

Magnesium Deficiency: Up to 80 Percent of Americans Are Magnesium-Deficient

There is also evidence that lack of magnesium may play a role in insomnia, and research indicates that a majority of Americans are magnesium deficient. One of the classic diagnostic symptoms of magnesium deficiency is insomnia, and low magnesium diets are consistently associated with poor sleep quality. [56] [57] [58] Magnesium deficient diets have been shown to significantly increase periods of wakefulness and decrease slow wave (restful) sleep. [59]

As you can see, micronutrients and especially unnatural light exposure can both have a powerful impact on our ability to sleep, and our sleep quality, in turn, is a major factor that determines how fat or lean we are—perhaps as important as nutrition.

---

56 Breakthroughs, N. (2009, September 8). "Insomnia: Studies Confirm Calcium And Magnesium Effective." Medical News Today. Retrieved from http://www.medicalnewstoday.com/releases/163169 .

57 Nielsen, F. H., Johnson, L. K., & Zeng, H. (2010). Magnesium supplementation improves indicators of low magnesium status and inflammatory stress in adults older than 51 years with poor quality sleep. Magnes Res. 23 (4), 158-68. doi: 10.1684/mrh.2010.0220.

58 Abbasi, B., Kimiagar, M., Sadeghniiat, K., Shirazi, M. M., Hedayati, M., & Rashidkhani, B. (2012). The effect of magnesium supplementation on primary insomnia in elderly: A double-blind placebo-controlled clinical trial. J Res Med Sci. 17(12), 1161-9.

59 Depoortere H, Françon D, Llopis J. (1993). Effects of a magnesium-deficient diet on sleep organization in rats. 27(4):237-45.

A Summary of the Neurological Causes of Increased Body Fat Set-Point

There are three main neurological causes of increased body fat set-point:

1. High food reward—this is processed food, particularly a combination of sugars and fats together. A high food reward diet progressively dissociates our eating behaviors from--and drives us to eat beyond--our actual biological need for fuel.
2. High food variety—this is exactly what it sounds like. Having an endless variety of options of highly rewarding foods available to us around every corner drives chronic overconsumption of calories and fat gain.
3. Circadian rhythm disruption—disrupted circadian rhythm is an often overlooked, but major cause of fat gain. It will cause fatigue, metabolism slowdown, and it will throw off normal appetite regulation and drive calorie overconsumption.

Now, if you combine all three of these neurological causes, you have a very potent recipe for fat gain.

The Neurological factors by themselves are massive, but we still have several other factors driving fat gain: The Cellular/Hormonal factors.

The Cellular / Hormonal Causes of Fat Gain

In order to understand what's going on at the cellular and hormonal levels that causes fat gain, let's first do a quick refresher on how the body fat set-point system works. The body fat set-point system works by just manipulating a couple of things—hunger/fullness and slowing or speeding up the metabolism. Hunger/fullness obviously controls how many calories you take in, and how fast your metabolism is controls how many calories your body burns. So just through those two things—hunger and metabolism—the body can almost completely regulate both your calorie intake and calorie expenditure for the purpose of making sure that calories in equal calories out and that your bodyweight stays stable over time.

Remember this graph:

The basic way that your body tries to keep a stable bodyweight:

	HUNGER	METABOLISM	RESULT
PERIOD OF OVEREATING	⬇	⬆	Bodyweight stays stable
PERIOD OF UNDEREATING	⬆	⬇	Bodyweight stays stable

Now, there is something very strange that happens in people who are overweight and obese. Given that they are *overconsuming* calories, you would expect them to have *fast metabolisms*. That's how the body fat set-point system works, remember? When you over-eat, hunger is supposed to go down and the metabolism is supposed to speed up.

But there's just one problem here: People who are overweight and obese virtually always have the opposite of what we would expect to see in a person who's overeating— they have lots of hunger, typically combined with a *slow* metabolism!

They have something called "leptin resistance," which throws off the balance of this system. Leptin is a hormone that is the focus of many obesity researchers, as many believe it is the key to understanding fat gain. Why? Leptin is a hormone secreted into the blood by fat cells, and its job is to let the brain know how much energy stores (body fat) it has and to modify calorie intake and metabolic rate accordingly. The more fat cells and the more full of fat those fat cells are, the more leptin you have in the blood—and the more it tells the brain, "Okay, we fat cells are all full of fat right now ... we've got plenty of energy ... so now, let's decrease our food intake and increase metabolic rate."

The less fat you have on your body, the less leptin you have in your blood, and the more it gives your brain the message, "Okay, we're running low on energy—time to eat some food, and if you don't find food, we'll have to slow down metabolic rate and decrease calorie burning so we don't burn off all our fuel stores." (Note: The system is more complex than this, and numerous other hormones and peptides are involved in the regulation of energy intake and metabolic rate, but for simplicity's sake, let's just focus on leptin, since it's the main one). In essence, low leptin signals to the brain "take in food and slow metabolic rate," and high leptin signals "take in less food and increase metabolic rate."

The "leptin resistance" that we find in overweight and obese people means that they do indeed have high levels of leptin (just as we would expect to see in people with lots of body fat), yet their brains don't seem to be responding to it in the way that we would expect.

In fact, their brains are not sensing the fact that there is an abundance of leptin and are responding in the same way the brain would respond to a situation in which the person is *undereating*. According to researchers Horvath and Gao, "When this feedback mechanism is disrupted, the brain continuously 'senses' a state of negative energy balance, promotes feeding, and reduces energy expenditure by default." [60] In other words, their brains aren't sensing all that leptin, so the brain actually responds to this situation as if there were very *low* levels of leptin—thus stimulating hunger and decreasing metabolic rate. As a result, **they exhibit all the typical symptoms we would expect to**

---

60 Gao, Q. & Horvath, T. L. (2008). Cross-talk between estrogen and leptin signaling in the hypothalamus. American Journal of Physiology - Endocrinology and Metabolism, 294, E817-E826. doi: 10.1152/ajpendo.00733.2007.

see in an anorexic person or a person suffering through a famine—they are constantly fatigued with low energy levels, they are often sensitive to cold, they are hungry very often, etc. **They are exhibiting all the symptoms of people who are starving of calories due to under-eating!**

Here's what researchers Horvath and Gao have to say on this fascinating paradox:

"Although obesity is a state in which a huge amount of excess body energy (fat) is accumulated, the behavior and physiology of obese individuals mirror those promoted during a state of negative energy balance, including hyperphagia and low metabolic rates. Under normal conditions, brain regions involved in long-term energy balance, by definition, must sense the amount of existing fuel in the body and use this knowledge to adjust energy intake and expenditure. That is, energy homeostasis is maintained tightly by surveillance of and responses to alteration in body energy stores: a negative energy balance promotes food intake and restricts energy expenditure, and vice versa... However, when leptin signaling is disrupted, as in leptin resistance or, in extreme cases, in leptin or leptin receptor deficiencies, the energy homeostatic machineries recognize a state of extreme negative energy balance and initiate various behavioral and physiological responses, regardless of actual body energy (fat) stores. Animals and humans with leptin signaling disrupted are not only hyperphagic but also have extreme difficulty utilizing stored energy." [61]

This is a very important fact. It's telling you that the cells of obese people are actually starving for energy (like an anorexic person, or someone in a famine), yet they are actually in a state of having a caloric overabundance (lots of body fat stores) well beyond their body's biological need.

This is a paradox: Obese people actually have an excess of energy in their bodies, but their biology is exhibiting the symptoms of cells chronically starved for energy.

---

61 Gao, Q. & Horvath, T. L. (2008). Cross-talk between estrogen and leptin signaling in the hypothalamus. American Journal of Physiology - Endocrinology and Metabolism, 294, E817-E826. doi: 10.1152/ajpendo.00733.2007.

I call this situation "The Metabolism Gap," because **there is now a discrepancy between the amount of calories being *taken in* and how many calories the body is actually *sensing* are present. There is a mismatch between how much you're eating and how much the cells are actually getting. You're eating a ton, but your cells are still somehow starving!**

Insulin resistance is one example of this sort of metabolic mismatch. Insulin resistance, as we all know, is characterized by an overabundance of sugar in the blood. This leads many to believe—very simplistically—that it's just a problem of "too much sugar." In reality, the blood does indeed have more sugar in it than a normal person, however, the *cells* are actually getting *less* sugar inside of them than what is considered normal and healthy (with lower blood sugar). This is what I'm talking about here—the gap between the amount of energy/calories actually present in the body and the amount of energy/calories that the cells are actually receiving.

If you understand this, one thing should become immediately obvious: The typical "burn more calories and eat fewer calories" approach to fat loss is actually trying to further *starve an already starving body!*

The mainstream approach to fat loss is calorie deprivation. Just deprive your body of calories by burning more calories than you take in, and you'll get fat loss, right?

The reason people who are overweight have such an awful time sticking to these regimens is not because they're lazy or have weak wills, it's because this strategy is actually further starving their already starving cells. So their biology fights against the regime with all its might, increasing hunger so they feel compelled to eat, destroying muscle instead of fat, causing extreme fatigue, *slowing their metabolism even more,* and predisposing them to future fat regain. They end up suffering as they try to starve themselves and force themselves to exercise even though they feel fatigued, but they just can't sustain the fight against their own biology. Biology always wins out.

If you understand all this, then the question is: What causes this mismatch between the amount of calories you're eating and the amount your cells are getting?

I believe that the major player here is *metabolic damage*.

Metabolic damage and the gap between the amount of energy actually present in the body vs. how much the cells are receiving is, based on my research, another major driver of the obesity epidemic.

Metabolic damage can come from a few different places:

1. METABOLICALLY TOXIC FOODS

What I mean by this is foods that actively decrease the amount of energy your cells are producing, and thus slow down your metabolism. Let me preface this section by saying that I almost hesitate to mention the notion of metabolically toxic foods at all, because many people have very black-and-white extreme responses to any food that they are told could be damaging to their health. Word gets out that "gluten is unhealthy" and we all of the sudden get a fad where everyone—including people who have no reaction to gluten—wants to go "gluten-free." A few diet gurus come saying that "sugar is toxic" or "insulin makes you fat" (both assertions based in pseudoscience) and everyone all of the sudden wants to go low-carb, and starts getting all crazy about avoiding sugar and carbs. (And then we have people running around thinking that sugar magically converts into fat in their bodies and we have nutrition gurus saying things like "it's not fat that makes you fat, it's carbs that turn into fat"). Given that we already have far too many diet gurus out there trying to give us a list of all the "forbidden foods," my goal here is not to create yet *another* list of forbidden foods for you to avoid at all costs and structure your diet around. **The whole frame of restriction and forbidden foods is a fundamentally flawed approach that sets people up for unhealthy and unnecessarily neurotic relationships with food. Rather than asking "what should I remove from my diet and avoid at all costs," a much better approach to nutrition is to ask "what are the ideal sources** of nutrients that support optimal cellular and metabolic function?" After you ask that question, then the goal is simply to go about making those foods the focus of your meals--NOT to develop an eating disorder while trying to follow some strict regimen of avoiding a long list of devil foods.

It is also important to note that I am *not* saying "all foods are equally good sources of nutrients—nothing is better or worse than anything else." There are most definitely foods which are better sources of nutrients than others, and there are some foods which can—at least, in some people—contribute to fat gain.

The point here is that you should *not* read this section and then think "so and so devil food is making me fat, and I must eliminate it from my diet." Among all of the different causes of fat gain that I am presenting in this book, consumption of metabolically toxic foods is a minor player in the overall scheme of things—it is not nearly as significant as almost every other factor listed in this book, like circadian rhythm disruption, highly rewarding foods, and the other cellular/hormonal factors you're going to read about in the next sections. So please do *not* read this section and then create a list of forbidden foods for yourself. Instead, I recommend structuring your meals around *intentionally* seeking out *ideal* sources of nutrients, not around avoidance of "bad foods."

Moreover, if you're someone who has a long history of trying and failing on excessively restrictive diets and you've developed eating disorders (like anorexia, bulimia, emotional eating, or binge eating disorder), you do NOT need any more rules around how you should eat--you may in fact, need to opposite in order to re-estabilish a healthy relationship with food. It's important that you start with a healthy relationship with food as a baseline before trying to adopt any dietary fat loss strategies. If this applies to you, please be aware that this book is not intended to treat or cure eating disorders--it is intended to teach the fundamental principles of lasting fat loss. For those who have disordered eating habits, there are many tools for those with eating disorders available--

books like _Intuitive Eating_, the numerous CBT (cognitive-behavioral therapy) and DBT (dialectical behavioral therapy) books, Matt Stone's _Diet Recovery_ 1 and 2, as well as psychotherapy are great places to get started. If you have an eating disorder (or severely disordered relationship with food) please take steps to address that through the tools above before trying to adopt any serious attempt at losing fat using nutritional modification.

Having given those disclaimers, I will however mention a few foods here that are things to be aware of, and that can cause problems for some people. There are several foods that are (or can be, in some people) metabolically toxic. Here are the most common culprits:

- **Excess Omega-6 Polyunsaturated Fats (PUFAs):** There are two major types of PUFAs—omega-3 and omega-6. Omega-3s are the ones we've all been hearing so much about in the news over the last few years. These come from foods like seafood and eggs (in the form DHA and EPA) and from seeds like flax and walnuts (in the less absorbable form ALA). Then we have the omega-6 fats, which are found in a wide-range of different foods, but are most concentrated in vegetable oils like canola oil, grape seed oil, corn oil, soy oil, and most nut/seed oils.

Most researchers believe that omega-6 and omega-3 intake should be balanced (estimates about the optimal ratio range from 1:1 to 5:1) and that if an inappropriate balance exists, this may predispose to various health woes. Here's where the problem comes in: Omega-6 consumption in the U.S. has skyrocketed in the last century, as we've been told by health authorities to avoid butter and saturated fat like the plague (since "they clog our arteries") and to replace those fats with "healthy" vegetable oils. Out with butter, in with margarine and canola oil. Out with steak and egg yolks, in with chicken and egg white omelets. As a result of this shift in thinking, we've seen intakes of omega-6 fats rise to levels well beyond anything that's ever occurred in human history, and these omega-6s have been piling up in our tissues.

Since the invention of vegetable oils, like canola oil, corn oil, sunflower oil, grape seed oil, and soy oil, roughly 100 years ago and the successful lobbying by vegetable oil corporations to incorporate these oils into the food supply, these oils have found their way into just about every processed food in existence—from store-bought sauces and dressings to virtually every kind of processed grain product, from chips to granola bars. If it's in a package, it's a good bet that it's full of vegetable oils. Nuts and seeds, as well as nut and seed oils/butters/milks—foods commonly used by health-conscious people—are also a huge source of omega-6 PUFAs. And, conventionally raised animal meats, like pork, farmed fish, eggs, and especially poultry, are chock-full of omega-6 PUFAs, unlike their naturally raised (grass-fed, free-range, and wild-caught) counterparts, which have far fewer omega-6 PUFAs. What's worse is that many people have been convinced that these oils are "healthy," and we're now using margarine (hydrogenated vegetable oils) instead of butter, and replacing old cooking fats, like butter and tallow, with the easily-oxidized canola oil and grape seed oil.

The concentration of these fats in our tissues has increased dramatically over the last few generations, and many different widely-respected nutrition gurus have blamed this extreme accumulation of omega-6 fats in our tissues (and the skewed omega-6 to omega-3 balance) for all sorts of modern health woes, from heart disease, to depression, to arthritis, to diabetes, to obesity. Numerous studies in fact have implicated these oils in increasing inflammation, intensifying the stress response, contributing to insulin resistance, and inhibiting thyroid hormone production. [62] [63] [64] [65] [66] [67] [68] [69] [70] [71] [72] [73] [74]

62 Central Committee for Medical and Community Program of the American Heart Association. (1961). Dietary fat and its relation to heart attacks and strokes. Journal of American Medical Association. 175, 389-391.

63 Harris, W. S., Mozaffarian, D., Rimm, E., Kris-Etherton, P., Rudel, L. L., Appel, L. J., … Sacks, F. (2009). Omega-6 fatty acids and risk for cardiovascular disease: A science advisory from the American Heart Association Nutrition Subcommittee of the Council on Nutrition, Physical Activity, and Metabolism; Council on Cardiovascular Nursing; and Council on Epidemiology and Prevention. Circulation, 119(6), 902- 907.

64 Masterjohn, C. (2008). How essential are the essential fatty acids? The PUFA report part i: A critical review of the requirement for polyunsaturated fatty acids. Cholesterol-And-Health.Com Special Reports, 1(2), 1-25.

65 Ziboh, V. A., & Hsia, S. L. (1972). Effects of prostaglandin E2 on rat skin: Inhibition of sterol ester biosynthesis and clearing of scaly lesions in essential fatty acid deficiency. J Lipid Res, 13, 458-466.

66 Ip, C., Carter, C. A., & Ip, M. M. (1985). Requirement of essential fatty acids for mammary tumorigenesis. Cancer Res. 45(5), 1997-2001.

67 Pearce, M. L. & Dayton, S. (1971). Incidence of cancer in men on a diet high in polyunsaturated fat, Lancet, 1, 464-467.

68 K. L. Erickson, et al., "Dietary lipid modulation of immune responsiveness," Lipids 18, 468-74, 1983

69 Erickson, K. L, Adams, D. A, & McNeill, C. J. (1983). Dietary lipid modulation of immune responsiveness. Lipids, 18, 468-74.

70 Osborne, T. B., & Mendel, L. B. (1920). Growth on diets poor in true fats. J Biol Chem. 45(1), 145-152

71 Ikemoto, S., Takahashi, M., Tsunoda, N., Maruyama, K., Itakura, H., & Ezaki, O. (1996). High-fat diet-induced hyperglycemia and obesity in mice: Differential effects of dietary oils. Metabolism, 45(12), 1539-46.

72 Jen, K. L, Buison, A., Pellizzon, M., Ordiz, F., Jr., Santa Ana, L., & Brown, J. (2003). Differential effects of fatty acids and exercise on body weight regulation and metabolism in female Wistar rats. Exp Biol Med (Maywood), 228(7), 843-9.

73 Massiera, F., Barbry, P., Guesnet, P., Joly, A., Luquet, S., Moreilhon-Brest, C.,… Ailhaud, G. A. (2010). Western-like fat diet is sufficient to induce a gradual enhancement in fat mass over generations. J Lipid Res. 51(8):2352-61. doi: 10.1194/jlr.M006866.

74 Hibbeln, J. R., Nieminen, L. RG., Blasbalg, T. L., Riggs, J. A. and Lands, W. EM. (2006). Healthy intakes of n−3 and n−6 fatty acids: Estimations

The research, however, is still not entirely clear on what the real health effects of these fats are, and for as many studies as we have showing ill effects from their consumption, we have others showing no deleterious effects. For every diet guru that cherry picks the studies to support the notion that vegetable oils are toxic, we have other studies showing that they don't cause any problems.[75]

One thing we do know is that these fats are most definitely not actively health-promoting and their consumption (along with the lowering of saturated fat intake) has certainly not helped prevent or treat the heart disease epidemic (or any other degenerative disease), like was originally claimed. Heart disease has skyrocketed the most in countries where omega-6 PUFA consumption is highest. In fact, there is actually one country in particular that provides a unique glimpse into the effects of higher polyunsaturated fat consumption, particularly from omega-6 fatty acids. Scientists are now referring to this as the "Israeli Paradox," because they have been shocked to discover that Israel, despite much higher consumption of the supposedly healthy and beneficial unsaturated fats than any other country, actually has much higher rates of the degenerative diseases that plague Western countries.

"Israel has one of the highest dietary polyunsaturated/saturated fat ratios in the world; the consumption of omega-6 polyunsaturated fatty acids (PUFA) is about 8% higher than in the USA, and 10-12% higher than in most European countries. In fact, Israeli Jews may be regarded as a population-based dietary experiment of the effect of a high omega-6 PUFA diet, a diet that until recently was widely recommended. Despite such national habits, there is paradoxically a high prevalence of cardiovascular diseases,

considering worldwide diversity. The American Journal of Clinical Nutrition, 83(6), S1483-1493S.

75 Guyenet, S. (2011). Seed oils and Body Fatness—A problematic Revisit. Retrieved from: http://wholehealthsource.blogspot.com/2011/08/seed-oils-and-body-fatness-problematic.html

hypertension, non-insulin-dependent diabetes mellitus and obesity-all diseases that are associated with hyperinsulinemia (HI) and insulin resistance (IR), and grouped together as the insulin resistance syndrome or syndrome X. There is also an increased cancer incidence and mortality rate, especially in women, compared with western countries. Studies suggest that high omega-6 linoleic acid consumption might aggravate HI and IR, in addition to being a substrate for lipid peroxidation and free radical formation. Thus, rather than being beneficial, high omega-6 PUFA diets may have some long-term side effects, within the cluster of hyperinsulinemia, atherosclerosis and tumorigenesis."[76]

To put all that in simple terms: Israelis have a much higher intake of omega-6 PUFAs than any other country, and, they have much *higher* rates of heart disease, diabetes, and cancer—the very conditions that we were told these oils were supposed to protect against. Is this direct causation, or some confounding factor? The truth is that we don't fully know yet. As it stands now with the current scientific data, it isn't fully clear exactly what the physiological effects of these oils are.

What *is* abundantly clear, however, is that omega 6 consumption has shot up dramatically in recent decades, and that **Americans (and most other modernized countries) are participating in a completely uncontrolled experiment that no one really knows the end result of.** Personally, I believe that this huge increase in omega-6 consumption represents a radical departure from the norms of the evolutionary diet, and I do think there is good reason to be concerned that it is a threat to our health. These oils have built up in our tissues dramatically in a very short period of time, and I believe that we will discover that there are indeed significant consequences to this. Though the consequences of this radical shift in our fatty acid intake will not likely be fully understood for another couple of decades.

---

76 Yam, D., Eliraz, A., & Berry, E. M. (1996). Diet and disease--the Israeli paradox: possible dangers of a high omega-6 polyunsaturated fatty acid diet. Isr J Med Sci, 32(11), 1134-43.

In the meantime, **if you don't wish to be a guinea pig in the completely uncontrolled experiment of extremely high omega-6 consumption** (which I believe is very likely to have metabolically toxic effects over time), I strongly advise dramatically lowering your intake of foods rich in omega-6 fatty acids. The research isn't conclusive yet, but I'm betting that the research will eventually confirm that vegetable oils are indeed metabolically toxic and unfit for human consumption.

- **Gluten:** Gluten is not universally toxic, and in truth, there are a great many people who do just fine with gluten and have no adverse reaction to it at all. For these people, going "gluten-free" is not likely to offer any profound health or fat loss benefits. However, there are also a significant number of people who do have negative health effects from eating gluten-containing foods and may not even realize that it's coming from gluten. Consuming gluten when you are intolerant to it can wreak havoc in the body and cause countless symptoms. Why? Simple: The way gluten wreaks havoc starts in the intestine by causing inflammation of the gut and leaky gut. This means that undigested food particles and toxins (like the potent endotoxin produced by bacteria in the gut) can then leak into your bloodstream. This causes a cascade of inflammation, immune system over-activity (potentially leading to autoimmune conditions), cellular damage, and overburdened organs (like the liver), which results in hormonal imbalance and an increase in stress hormones. This situation is toxic to every physiological system in your body, from the hormonal to the cellular level.

As I said, not everyone reacts to gluten, but it's also important to recognize that 1 in 8 people who have celiac disease are not aware of it. So if you suspect that you may have a bad reaction to it, or you're experiencing unexplained symptoms of some kind, it's a good idea to get tested by your doctor to check your reaction to gluten, and/or get gluten out of your diet completely for a period of time to figure out if the symptoms you are experiencing (fat gain, fatigue, inflammation, low levels of youth hormones, autoimmune problems, hypothyroidism, etc.) are coming from this substance.

- **Micronutrient Absorption-Blocking Foods:** Certain foods can effectively function as *anti-nutrients*. That is, they are not only not supplying nutrients to your body, but they are actively *blocking* your body from taking in vitamins and minerals. By blocking the absorption of various micronutrients, these foods--which include grains, legumes, and nuts/seeds--can potentially contribute to micronutrient deficiencies, which in turn, are a significant contributor to low metabolic rate. When the cells are deprived of adequate levels of things like calcium, magnesium, vitamin A, copper, selenium, zinc, and other micronutrients, the cells are not able to produce energy efficiently. **Having said that, this is an extremely minor factor with weak supporting evidence that these anti-nutrients are a major factor in poor health or the obesity epidemic.**

I am choosing to intentionally not elaborate on the science on this topic for a few important reasons that I want to emphasize: It is, by far, the *least* important aspect in this book, as micronutrient deficiencies arise primarily because of eating foods poor in micronutrient content--not because of anti-nutrients. 2) These foods have been demonized ad nauseaum by many Paleo gurus. 3) My goal with this book is to get you to frame your approach to food as "how can I choose foods richer in nutrients?"rather than "how can I avoid _____ devil foods?" so I don't want to add more fuel to fire of food avoidance.

If you're someone who habitually derives a *very large* portion of your diet from unsoaked grains, nuts/seeds, and legumes, it can potentially result in problems. And you may benefit from minimizing your consumption of these foods. But there is likely nothing to worry about if you eat these foods in moderation. If you do consume grains, legumes, and nuts/seeds as a large part of your diet, properly preparing these foods is a smart idea to avoid problems. You can read on that subject <u>HERE</u> and <u>HERE</u>.

- **Trans-fats:** Most people have heard about trans-fats by now, so I won't belabor the point. These are generally hydrogenated or heated vegetable oils. Margarine, or the partially hydrogenated oils found in tons of packaged foods, and highly heated vegetable oils (like canola oil used in cooking, for example) are the major sources here. They are chemically altered and unnatural fats which are genuinely very toxic to our bodies. Due to our consumption of packaged foods that contain hydrogenated oils, our consumption of fried foods, and cooking in vegetable oils, Americans on the standard American diet eat roughly 4-7% of their daily calories as trans-fats, which is not good. Trans-fats are bad news, and they're linked with lots of different health issues, from heart disease to diabetes to Alzheimer's. This isn't even controversial anymore, and several scientists have now been very vocal about getting them banned from the food supply. Eliminate them from your diet!

- **Pesticides/Herbicides/Plastic Softeners:** We don't yet have complete answers in the research about the effects of pesticides and herbicides used in conventional farming, or of things like BPA (and other plastic softening chemicals). But we do know that many of these chemicals can be endocrine (i.e. hormonal) disruptors in humans— specifically, they tend to be estrogen promoting. BPA (a chemical commonly found in plastics and canned foods) is known to produce damaging hormonal effects even in very small doses.[77] [78]It's too early to conclusively say that this is a major factor driving fat gain, but in general, I believe there is already enough evidence to suggest that we should not be consuming foods and drinks out of plastic containers, and we should be eating organic produce and naturally-raised animal foods.

- **Allergens:** This is an individual thing as each person has different foods they are more or less allergic to. Consuming any food you're allergic to causes a cascade of inflammation, oxidative damage, stress hormones, and an immune reaction in your body. All of these decrease the ability of your cells to produce energy efficiently and thus cause the metabolism to slow down.

Please be aware that I'm most definitely not blaming the entire obesity epidemic on just vegetable oils, trans-fats, and BPA. I do think that for many people, these things can be a significant contributing factor—vegetable oils, in particular, and gluten (for those sensitive to it)—but these substances are just one of numerous different causes of fat gain. If anything, these are likely *minor* contributors to fat gain relative to the other causes mentioned in this book. However, one important point to recognize is that something which has toxins in it may not be a problem at all in small amounts (e.g. a little vegetable oils here and there), but when you start eating lots of these foods, and *combining lots of these foods,* on a daily basis for years or decades, the toxic effects add up. In other words, if the *majority* of your daily diet is composed of foods with vegetable oils, soy products, unsprouted grains/nuts/seeds/legumes, foods packaged in cans or plastics with BPA, and transfats, you're eventually gonna run

---

77 vom Saal FS, Nagel SC, Timms BG, Welshons WV. (2005). Implications for human health of the extensive bisphenol A literature showing adverse effects at low doses: a response to attempts to mislead the public. Toxicology. 2005 Sep 1;212(2-3):244-52

78 Hormonally Active Agents in the Environment. Retrieved from:
   http://www.nap.edu/openbook.php?isbn=0309064198

into trouble on that program. And by trouble, I mean that it's likely to contribute to making you sick and fat.

Relative to the other factors driving fat gain that I talk about in this book, metabolically toxic foods is a minor one. So please don't fixate on creating a list of forbidden foods for yourself! Food reward, micronutrient-deficiencies that arise from processed food consumption, and circadian rhythm disruption (and the factors you're about to learn about) are much more dominant factors in driving fat gain than any specific harmful foods.

Why Carbohydrates/Sugar Didn't Make This List of Metabolically Toxic Foods—They Are Not Metabolically Toxic and They Are Not a Major Cause of Fat Gain

One thing you may have noticed that's rather conspicuously lacking from my list of metabolically toxic foods is the very thing that many popular nutrition gurus today commonly blame the entire obesity epidemic on: carbohydrates. Or perhaps more true to how these nutrition teachers usually portray it: carbohydrates, insulin, and sugar.

Many low-carb advocates—most notably, Gary Taubes—have promoted a hypothesis of obesity/fat gain known as "The Carbohydrate Theory of Obesity" that speculates that carbohydrates, sugar, and insulin have all sorts of metabolically toxic effects and put the body into a "fat-storing" hormonal state. (i.e., "Insulin is a fat storing hormone, and the more often we spike it by eating carbs, the more fat we become.")

Unfortunately, these claims (which are rather poor excuses for science) have gained considerable popularity, and it is now common to hear various nutrition "authorities" citing sugar consumption and insulin as the reasons why people get fat.

It is a shame that we even have to deal with this sort of pseudoscience in our day and age, since the Carbohydrate/Insulin Theory of Obesity has not been taken seriously by virtually any obesity scientist on the planet in over two decades. This theory was already proven wrong in numerous scientific studies and had been discarded by obesity and metabolism scientists by the late 1980s. The theory is just wrong, but largely due to ignorance of the science on the subject, many popular nutrition gurus today still promote low-carb myths and all sorts of carbohydrate and insulin-related pseudoscience.

If you would like to read more on this important issue, please check out my book _The Low Carb Myth_ which is an in-depth analysis of all the science around carbohydrates and insulin.

A common refrain to the assertion that carbohydrate consumption is not the cause (or even _a cause_) of fat gain is "Well, then how come me/my brother/my sister/my mom/my friend lost weight when we went low-carb?" Simple: It has nothing do with carbohydrate restriction—it has to do with the simple fact that most low-carb (especially low-carb Paleo) diets transition people to a diet that includes significantly more protein, significantly less processed foods, and more whole foods. Higher intake of whole foods and higher protein intake are both—in and of themselves—known to cause a spontaneous reduction in _total calorie intake_ of hundreds of calories per day. People lose weight not due to anything related to insulin or carbohydrates, but simply due to higher protein intake and higher whole food intake driving down their total daily calorie intake. The same exact weight loss can be seen on high-carbohydrate diets that include equal amounts of protein and whole foods. Research has indeed confirmed this, as I explained in the "Calories Do Matter, But You Should Not Count Them" section.[79]

The only things that very low-carb diets typically accomplish are creating unnecessary deprivation, cultivating obsessive-compulsive eating habits, teaching people to fight against and feel guilty about their carbohydrate cravings, perpetuating nutritional myths and ignorance, and causing hormonal and metabolic problems in the long term.

---

79 Soenen, S., Bonomi, A. G., Lemmens, S. G., Scholte, J., Thijssen, M. A., van Berkum, F., & Westerterp-Plantenga, M. S. (2012). Relatively high-protein or 'low-carb' energy-restricted diets for body weight loss and body weight maintenance?. Physiol Behav. 107(3):374-80. doi: 10.1016/j.physbeh.2012.08.004.

(Side note: Most of my clients come to me after years of strict low-carb eating wanting to fix all of the problems they've caused themselves from this way of eating, and much of my work now revolves around undoing the metabolic/hormonal damage that the low-carb diet fad is causing people. The most common problem of long-term low-carb dieters is hypothyroidism, which is rather significant, since thyroid hormone is the main regulator of the metabolism.)

Total calorie intake—not carbohydrates or insulin levels—dictates fat loss results. People who got results on low-carb diets have simply confused their carbohydrate avoidance with the spontaneous reduction in total calorie intake that occurs when someone eats a diet higher in protein and whole foods.

(A quick note for clarification: Some people may get confused at the above statement that calories do matter since I have previously stated that *forced calorie deprivation* is a very counterproductive approach to fat loss. To be clear, calories do matter. But there is a big difference between *deliberate and forced* calorie restriction (not a good thing) vs. a spontaneous and non-conscious reduction in calorie intake (a very beneficial thing). One of them creates fat loss which is against the body's will and inevitably results in failure in the long run, and the other creates fat loss which is in line with the body's will, which is critical for lasting success. Big difference. Also, do not mistake my previous berating of *forced calorie deprivation* as equating to "calories do not matter." There is nothing wrong with dietary strategies that act to unconsciously drive down total calorie intake—such as eating whole foods or having a higher protein intake—and these are actually very useful fat loss strategies. They are in fact, the major factors responsible for the few people who do get lasting success from changing their diet. I do not have a problem with this at all. I do however, have a problem with mistaking this spontaneous decrease in total calories consumed—that resulted from increased whole food and protein intake—with some magical effect of low-carb dieting. The fat was lost from the increased whole foods and protein intake, not anything to do with carbohydrates or insulin).

Having said that the carbohydrate/insulin theory of fat gain is bunk, it is worth noting that refined sugars—especially in the form of processed foods, where sugars are typically combined with fats and wrapped into a tasty artificial flavoring-laced treat—can absolutely contribute to neurologically driving calorie overconsumption via food reward. However, this is *not* due to carbohydrates or sugars *per se*. This is due to commercially prepared and professionally engineered food designed to maximize food reward. As Guyenet explains in the above article, cultures that consume massive amounts of whole-food carbohydrates and natural sugars, well beyond the paltry 50% carbohydrate diet Americans consume—like the Kitavans (69% carbohydrate diet), or the Okinawans (85% carbohydrate diet), or the Tukisenta and Ewe tribes (over 90% carbohydrate diet)—have negligible to nonexistent rates of obesity. The Tukisenta and Ewe tribes basically eat nothing but sweet potatoes and are spiking their insulin on huge scale after every meal, day after day, for decades. Yet these tribes remain perfectly lean despite constantly spiking this "fat storing" hormone insulin. But, take one of these tribes eating a predominantly carbohydrate diet and introduce them to Western processed foods, like has been done in many places in the world—for example, the Pima Indians—and you get an obesity epidemic. The traditional Pima diet was a high-carbohydrate diet consisting of beans, corn and squash, with wild fish, game meat and plants. *"Researchers at the NIDDK in Phoenix have estimated that the traditional Pima diet took about 70 percent of its calories in the form of carbohydrates, 15 percent in protein, and 15 percent in fat. By the 1950's (after the introduction of Western processed food) the proportions had changed to 61 percent carbohydrate, 15 percent in protein, and 24 percent in fat. In 1971 it was 44 percent carbohydrate, 12 percent protein, and 44 percent fat – a tripling of the fat content."* [80] During that span of time, the Pima have become the most obese and

---

80 Pool, R. (2000). Fat: Fighting the Obesity Epidemic. Oxford University Press.

diabetic population on the planet. The Pima Indians do not support the notion that "carbohydrates/insulin make you fat"— they show us that a diet based on *processed foods* makes you fat. [81] [82]

This (along with the many other lines of evidence Guyenet examines in the above article) clearly demonstrates that fat gain has nothing to do with insulin or carbohydrates or sugars *per se*. The nutritional causes of fat gain have to do primarily with *processed foods* and *food reward*, not carbohydrates or insulin.

Takeaway message: Contrary to much popular pseudoscience, carbohydrates and insulin are not major players in the obesity epidemic. In fact, carbohydrates are actually wonderful allies in your efforts to achieve your health and fat loss goals. Do not forcibly try to restrict your carbohydrate intake or fight your carbohydrate cravings. Just make sure to get them (like all other nutrients, such as fat and protein) only from *whole, unprocessed* foods.

2. CHRONIC CALORIE OVERCONSUMPTION

Perhaps the biggest metabolically toxic factor of all—much more so than the specific foods mentioned above—is chronic calorie overconsumption itself. Yes, the very thing that is created from all of these factors that drive up the body fat set-point, chronic overconsumption of calories, is extremely toxic to your

81 Smith, C. J., Nelson, R. G., Hardy, S. A., Manahan, E. M., Bennett, P. H., & Knowler, W. C. (1996). Survey of the diet of Pima Indians using quantitative food frequency assessment and 24-hour recall. Diabetic renal disease study. J Am Diet Assoc, 96(8), 778-84

82 Schulz, L. O., Bennett, P. H., Ravussin, E., Kidd, J. R., Kidd, K. K., Esparza, J., & Valencia, M. E. (2006). Effects of traditional and western environments on prevalence of type 2 diabetes in Pima Indians in Mexico and the U.S. Diabetes Care, 29(8), 1866-71.

cells.[83][84] To be clear, this is *not* about any specific nutrient (fats, proteins, or carbohydrates) as *all* nutrients become toxic to the cells when there is a chronic excess of nutrients in the blood.

We actually are built with a system wired into our biology that is designed to regulate concentrations of glucose and fatty acids in our blood, and mop up any excess by storing it away in fat cells. So how do we actually get toxic effects on our cells from overconsumption of calories if we have fat cells designed to mop up any calorie excess? Well, as we accumulate body fat, our fat cells begin to do this job less and less effectively,[85] thus leaving an excess of nutrients in the bloodstream and creating toxic effects on the cells. This is in fact the major cause of insulin resistance (type II diabetes).[86] Chronic calorie overconsumption creates a situation where the cells intentionally become less efficient at taking in nutrients and producing cellular energy, since they are trying to protect themselves from the toxicity of the chronic overabundance of nutrients in the blood. [87] This is somewhat of a vicious cycle—things that drive chronic calorie overconsumption cause you to be fat, and that increased body

---

83 Hoehn, K. L, Salmon, A. B., Hohnen-Behrens, C., Turner, N., Hoy, A. J., Maghzal, J. G., & Jamesa, D. E. (2009). Insulin resistance is a cellular antioxidant defense mechanism. Proc Natl Acad Sci U S A. 106(42), 17787–17792. doi: 10.1073/pnas.0902380106.

84 Mittendorfer, B., Magkos, F., Fabbrini, E., Mohammed, B. S., & Klein, S. (2009). Relationship between body fat mass and free fatty acid kinetics in men and women. Obesity (Silver Spring). 17(10),1872-7. doi: 10.1038/oby.2009.224.

85 Mitrou, P., Boutati, E., Lambadiari, V., Maratou, E., Komesidou, V., Papakonstantinou, A., … Dimitriadis, G. (2010). Rates of lipid fluxes in adipose tissue in vivo after a mixed meal in morbid obesity. Int J Obes (Lond). 34(4), 770-4. doi: 10.1038/ijo.2009.293.

86 Guyenet, S. (2012, January 6). What causes insulin resistance? Part I. Retrieved from http://wholehealthsource.blogspot.com/2011/11/what-causes-insulin-resistance-part-i.html .

87 Hoehn, K. L., Salmon, A. B., Hohnen-Behrens, C., Turner, N., Hoy, A. J., Maghzal, G. J., Stocker, R., … Jamesa, D. E. (2009). Insulin resistance is a cellular antioxidant defense mechanism. Proc Natl Acad Sci U S A. 106(42), 17787–17792. doi: 10.1073/pnas.0902380106.

fatness itself then contributes to a state of physiology (the cellular toxicity of chronic nutrient excess) which contributes to further fat gain.

3. FORCED CALORIE DEPRIVATION (i.e. most mainstream approaches to fat loss)

As I have explained previously, chronically trying to force your body into a situation where it is burning more calories than it takes in is *counterproductive*. It causes short-term weight loss, then fat regain, and it typically causes muscle destruction and metabolism slowdown. This approach is flawed at its foundation, because it tries to further starve cells that are already starving for energy. **Do you see the irony here? The very thing that everyone is telling you to do if you want to lose fat—forcibly deprive your body of calories—is actually *contributing* to fat gain in the long term.** It is a very insidious trap that few people can actually see, because in the short term, calorie deprivation does appear to work for fat loss. So when people start gaining all the fat back, it is virtually always blamed on the individual. "Oh, well, you just didn't have enough willpower to continue the exercise and diet program." Wrong! The problem is not that the person didn't have the willpower to force themselves to continue depriving his or her body of calories, it's that they were put her on a program where they were fighting against their own biology, and eventually their biology won out. Biology always wins in the long term, as it can cause as much of a decrease in calories out as it needs to in order to fight against your attempts to starve it of calories. It will decrease thyroid hormone, destroy muscle mass, lower levels of other youth hormones, decrease your cells' sensitivity to thyroid hormone, decrease NEAT, and anything else it can to *decrease* the amount of energy your cells are using up. To recap: Forced calorie deprivation brought on by restricting food intake and burning tons of calories with exercise results in short-term weight loss, followed by metabolic damage (your metabolism slows down), and then fat regain. Combine that calorie restriction with hours of steady state cardio—a type of activity known to contribute to hypothyroidism and a slow metabolism[88] [89] [90]— and you have a potent recipe for priming your body for fat gain. Usually after a period of forced calorie deprivation, you don't just regain the fat you lost, but you regain more—piling layers on top of what you already had to begin with. According to a recent meta-analysis done at UCLA, dieting is, in fact, the single most powerful predictor of future weight gain— that is, forced calorie deprivation causes your set-point to go up over time. Here are some highlights from the landmark research conducted by these UCLA researchers:[91]

- "You can initially lose 5 to 10 percent of your weight on any number of diets, but then the weight comes back," said Traci Mann, UCLA associate professor of psychology and lead author of the study. "We found that the majority of people regained all the weight, plus more. Sustained weight loss was found only in a small minority of participants, while complete weight regain was found in the majority. Diets do not lead to sustained weight loss or health benefits for the majority of people."

- "Several studies indicate that dieting is actually a consistent predictor of future weight gain," said Janet Tomiyama, a co-author of the study.

- "What happens to people on diets in the long run?" Mann asked. "Would they have been better off to not go on a

88 Hackney, A., Dobridge, J. (2009). Thyroid hormones and the interrelationship of cortisol and prolactin: influence of prolonged, exhaustive exercise. Endokrynol Pol. 2009 Jul-Aug;60(4):252-7.

89 Beyleroglu, M. (2011). The effects of maximal aerobic exercise on cortisol and thyroid hormones in male field hockey players. African Journal of Pharmacy and Pharmacology Vol. 5(17), pp. 2002-2006.

90 Boyden TW, Pamenter RW, Rotkis TC, Stanforth P, Wilmore JH. Thyroidal changes associated with endurance training in women. Med Sci Sports Exerc. 1984 Jun;16(3):243-6.

91 Dieting Does Not Work, UCLA Researchers Report. Retrieved from: http://newsroom.ucla.edu/releases/Dieting-Does-Not-Work-UCLA-Researchers-7832?RelNum=7832

diet at all? We decided to dig up and analyze every study that followed people on diets for two to five years. We concluded most of them would have been better off not going on the diet at all. Their weight would be pretty much the same, and their bodies would not suffer the wear and tear from losing weight and gaining it all back."

- In a study where dieting obese people were followed for varying lengths of time, they had some very interesting findings: Among those who were followed for fewer than two years, 23 percent gained back more weight than they had lost, while of those who were followed for at least two years, 83 percent gained back more weight than they had lost. According to Mann, another study they analyzed found that 50 percent of dieters weighed more than 11 pounds over their starting weight five years after the diet.

- The researchers also pointed out that there is now solid scientific evidence suggesting that repeatedly losing and gaining weight is linked to cardiovascular disease, stroke, diabetes, and altered immune function.

- According to Tomiyama, "We asked what evidence is there that dieting works in the long term, and found that the evidence shows the opposite."

4. MACRONUTRIENT AND MICRONUTRIENT DEFICIENCIES

The processed foods-packed SAD (standard American diet) is a micronutrient deficient diet. It is deficient in countless vitamins and minerals, which are essential to your cells' ability to produce energy—that is, essential to a fast metabolism. In addition, many of the commonly advocated fad diets in recent decades actively cause metabolic damage. Low-fat diets can. Low-carb diets absolutely can. And vegan/vegetarian diets can. When you have a deficiency in either carbs, fat (the right kinds), or protein, in the long term it will cause significant metabolic damage. Vegans and vegetarians are often met with huge improvements in health after they shift to veganism/vegetarianism from the SAD (standard

American diet), and they are immediately convinced that veganism/vegetarianism is the holy grail for how it initially made them feel. What they don't realize is that this feeling has little to do with animal protein avoidance and much more to do with the benefits of eating a pure whole-foods diet based on fruits and vegetables. The same exact thing is true of low-carb diets. Low-carb diets can result in dramatic improvements in health after people shift from the SAD to going Paleo or low-carb, but what they don't realize is that these benefits have absolutely *nothing* to do with carbohydrate avoidance and everything to do with the fact that they shifted to eating a diet based on unrefined whole foods, dramatically lowering their intake of most of the metabolically-toxic foods I listed above. This is all good and well, except for just one thing: In the long term, both low-protein intake (or deficient amino acid profiles) from vegetarianism/veganism, and especially carbohydrate avoidance, actually *cause* metabolic dysfunction. Vegan and vegetarian diets typically lead to myriad micronutrient deficiencies.[92] [93] [94] [95] Low-carb diets have been proven to lower thyroid hormone in the long

---

92 Craig, W. J. (2010). Nutrition concerns and health effects of vegetarian diets. Nutr Clin Pract. 25(6), 613-20. doi: 10.1177/0884533610385707.

93 Rosell, M. S., Lloyd-Wright, Z., Appleby, P. N., Sanders, T. A. B., Allen, N. E., & Key, T. J. (2005). Long-chain n–3 polyunsaturated fatty acids in plasma in British meat-eating, vegetarian, and vegan men. Am J Clin Nutr. 82(2), 327-334.

94 Hunt, J. R. (2003). Bioavailability of iron, zinc, and other trace minerals from vegetarian diets. Am J Clin Nutr. 78 (3), 633S-639S.

95 Watanabe, F., Katsura, H., Takenaka, S., Fujita, T., Abe, K., Tamura, Y., … Nakano, Y. (1999). Pseudovitamin B(12) is the predominant cobamide of an algal health food, spirulina tablets. J Agric Food Chem. 47(11), 4736-41.

term and significantly slow down the metabolism.[96] [97] [98] [99] Common symptoms experienced by low-carb dieters are hormonal imbalance, low energy, fatigue, lack of motivation, sensitivity to cold, poor mood, hair loss, low libido, and many others. I have suffered many of these myself as I personally did strict low-carb Paleo eating for over a decade.

5. MOVEMENT DEFICIENCY AND EXCESSIVE SITTING

The final cellular/hormonal cause of fat gain relates to movement. Let me preface this section by making a critical distinction that most people have never even heard of: The distinction between *movement* and exercise. As you're about to find out, these are very different things—completely distinct factors in fact, that need to be separated out to be understood properly.

Believe it or not, lack of exercise does *not* appear to be a major factor in the obesity epidemic. Here's Guyenet on the matter: "Although I believe that exercise is part of a healthy lifestyle, and can help prevent fat gain and to some degree treat overweight, it probably can't explain the recent increase in fat mass in modern nations (i.e. the obesity epidemic). This is because exercise doesn't appear to have declined. There are various other possible explanations, such as industrial pollutants, a lack of sleep and psychological stress, which may play a role. But I feel that diet is

---

96 Hendler, R. G., Walesky, M., & Sherwin, R. S. (1986). Sucrose substitution in prevention and reversal of the fall in metabolic rate accompanying hypocaloric diets. Am J Med. 81(2), 280-4.

97 Mathieson RA, et al. The effect of varying carbohydrate content of a very-low-caloric diet on resting metabolic rate and thyroid hormones. Metabolism, May, 1986; 35 (5): 394-398.

98 Hendler, R. G., Walesky, M., & Sherwin, R. S. (1986). Sucrose substitution in prevention and reversal of the fall in metabolic rate accompanying hypocaloric diets. Am J Med. 81(2), 280-4.

99 Fery, F., Bourdoux, P., Christophe, J., & Balasse, E. O. (1982). Hormonal and metabolic changes induced by an isocaloric isoproteinic ketogenic diet in healthy subjects. Diabete Metab. 8(4), 299-305.

likely to be the primary cause (of the obesity epidemic)."[100] (Note: parentheses are mine).

To put it simply, the NHANES survey (US CDC National Health and Nutrition Examination Survey) from 1975 to 2006 shows us that over this span of time—roughly coinciding with the obesity epidemic—the number of sedentary people has actually gone *down* from 50% to 24%. **In other words, most of us are exercising *more*, not less, than we did 40 or 50 years ago.** This is the reason that lack of exercise is just not a very big factor that drives fat gain. If it was a major factor, we should've seen exercise go down, not up, during the last 50 years. Thus, as Guyenet states: "... I do think we can safely rule out inactivity as the reason we've gotten fatter. **In my mind, this only leaves one major possible cause for the obesity epidemic: changes in diet.** Don't get me wrong, I think exercise is good. It has numerous positive effects on physical and mental health. But it's not as powerful of a tool for fat loss and general health as diet...The reason is simple: the problems a person corrects with a good diet are caused by a poor diet to begin with." [101]

Guyenet is right—it's true that **people don't become fat due to a deficiency in Crossfit or P90X workouts. Thus trying to solve the problem by approaching it as a matter of adding in intense workouts to your life is not likely to get you very far.**

However, where Guyenet errs in my opinion is failing to adequately distinguish between exercise and *not moving*. He equates "inactivity" with "lack of exercise." These are not the same thing. Lack of exercise—i.e. gym workouts—is indeed not

---

100 Guyenet, S. (2010, January 23). The body fat setpoint, part III: Dietary causes of obesity. Retrieved from http://wholehealthsource.blogspot.com/2010/01/body-fat-setpoint-part-iii-dietary.html

101 Guyenet, S. (2010, January 23). The body fat setpoint, part III: Dietary causes of obesity. Retrieved from http://wholehealthsource.blogspot.com/2010/01/body-fat-setpoint-part-iii-dietary.html

a major factor in the obesity epidemic. **But too much *sitting* and lack of movement is most definitely a huge factor!** In fact, as you're about to find out, another prominent obesity scientist believes that it may just be the single most important factor.

Nutrition is unquestionably a massive factor driving the epidemic of fat gain we've seen over the last 50 years. However, it isn't everything. I believe that almost everyone out there who's in search of fat loss is so myopically fixated on *diet* and *exercise*, that they are overlooking a factor that is a huge piece of the fat loss puzzle: Non-exercise movement. (a.k.a. Non-exercise activity thermogenesis, or NEAT).

What is NEAT? It's basically all the movement that you do throughout the day as a natural result of simply living your life. It is *not* the stuff you do when you go to the gym like aerobics classes, riding the spin bike, or lifting weights. (Nor is it *just* fidgeting and twiddling your thumbs, as some mistakenly believe). NEAT encompasses all of the little movements of simply living our life—it's fidgeting, but also washing the car, running errands, climbing the stairs, walking down the street to the store, and even things like chewing gum and typing on your computer.

How important is NEAT? Well, obesity expert Dr. James Levine of the Mayo Clinic, goes so far as to state in his book *Move a Little, Lose a Lot* that he believes that too much sitting and lack of movement is *the* major cause of fat gain. In his words, **"Our current obesity and related health woes stem from the fact that modern life in the Internet-driven electronic age has increasingly leeched NEAT from our existence to the tune of up to 1,500 to 2,000 calories a day. And that loss is literally sucking the life out of us**...It's ironic, isn't it? You spend all day sitting, which should leave you with energy to burn by the end of the day. Yet you feel completely and utterly spent and wanting nothing more than to collapse when you get home."[102]

---

102 Levine, J. (2009). Move a Little, Lose a Lot. Crown Archetype.

Think about that for a moment. We have lost a whopping 1,500 to 2,000 calories per day from lack of NEAT. That's massive! Many people only take in and burn 1,300 or 1,500 *total* in a day—even after doing an hour workout at the gym! Optimal NEAT habits can literally *double* the baseline level of calories that our set-point system is regulating our energy balance (calories in-calories out). And poor NEAT habits can dramatically lower it. Think for a moment, about how this massive reduction in calorie burning affects our ability to stay lean. Indeed, we already know that there is a link between how much a person moves throughout the day and how fat or lean they are—lean people tend to stand and move for several more hours of the day, while obese people generally tend to stand for several less hours, and sit for several more hours each day.[103]

Dr. Levine, perhaps the world's foremost authority on NEAT, says that we humans now have an energy crisis—a human energy crisis. What is this crisis all about? Well I'll let him explain: "As a doctor who has spent more than twenty years studying human movement, obesity, and metabolism, I can tell you that **the way we are living and the way many of us are going about weight loss is absolutely, fundamentally wrong. Fifty years ago, there were no gyms; people rarely 'exercised,' and very few people struggled with being overweight. We managed our weight effortlessly because *we moved*. Now we struggle with it daily because we are desk sentenced."**[104]

Believe it or not, NEAT is actually significantly *more* important than our exercise habits when it comes to fat loss, yet virtually no one is talking about it. And it's not just of critical importance when it comes to fat loss, but also for health, vitality, avoiding diabetes and many other chronic diseases, enhancing energy

---

103 Johannsen DL, Welk GJ, Sharp RL, Flakoll PJ. Differences in daily energy expenditure in lean and obese women: the role of posture allocation. Obesity (Silver Spring). Jan 2008;16(1):34-39. - See more at: http://www.brinkzone.com/articles/a-neat-way-to-fat-loss/#sthash.NXe1XKsM.dpuf

104 Levine, J. (2009). Move a Little, Lose a Lot. Crown Archetype.

levels, speeding up our metabolism, and even has a huge impact on how long we live.

Most of us don't realize it because we weren't around to see it, but our ancestors lived a very active life that entailed minimal amounts of sitting and tons of daily walking (most studies indicate between four to ten miles per day on average). This was the norm for our species for hundreds of thousands of years. Yet, just over the last few decades, there has been a radical departure from that way of life. Today, we live in a totally new kind of world—a new kind of lifestyle where we do minimal amounts of standing, minimal amounts of walking, and many of us spend twelve to fifteen hours a day sitting on our butts. **We are guinea pigs in a totally new experiment that has never before been conducted in human history**, and we are just starting to see the scientific data about the results of this little experiment. Sitting is now linked with:

- **Shortened lifespan:** One study, published in the British Journal of Sports Medicine, which included nearly 12,000 Australian adults, concluded that each hour spent watching television after the age of 25 reduces your life expectancy by nearly 22 minutes. To give you a reference for comparison of just how significant that is, when the authors compared that reduction to smoking, they found that each cigarette reduces your life expectancy only by about 11 minutes. The researchers found that adults who spend an average of six hours a day sitting in front of the TV will reduce their life expectancy by just under five years, compared to someone who does not watch TV.

- **Increased risk of heart disease, type II diabetes, and many cancers:** Research now indicates that sitting for several hours each day is as significant a health risk factor as obesity and smoking. Many studies show increased mortality from heart disease and diabetes in those who sit frequently, and some studies even suggest that excessive sitting is responsible for over 150,000 cases of cancer each year. [105] [106] [107] [108] [109] [110] Another meta-analysis that compiled the data from 18 studies that in total included nearly 800,000 people, found that those who sat for the longest periods of time were twice as likely to have diabetes or heart disease compared to those who sat the least.[111] (This, of course, could just be confusing correlation with causation. Yet, when we look at the immediate effects on cellular health of even a few hours of sitting, the picture becomes clearer).

---

105 Mark, A. E. & Janssen, I. (2008). Relationship between screen time and metabolic syndrome in adolescents. J Public Health. 30 (2), 153-160. doi: 10.1093/pubmed/fdn022.

106 Saunders, T. (2012). Excessive sitting lowering US life expectancy by ~2 years. Retrieved from http://blogs.plos.org/obesitypanacea/2012/07/10/excessive-sitting-lowering-us-life-expectancy-by-2-years/?utm_source=feedburner&utm_medium=feed&utm_campaign=Feed%3A+plos%2Fblogs%2Fobesitypanacea+%28Blogs+-+Obesity+Panacea%29&utm_content=Google+Reader

107 Veerman, J. L., Healy, G. N., Cobiac, L. J., Vos, T., Winkler, E. A. H., Owen, N., & Dunstan, D. W. (2012). Television viewing time and reduced life expectancy: a life table analysis. Br J Sports Med. 46, 927-930 doi:10.1136/bjsports-2011-085662

108 Veerman, J. L., Healy, G. N., Cobiac, L. J., Vos, T., Winkler, E. A., Owen, N., & Dunstan, D. W. (2012). Television viewing time and reduced life expectancy: a life table analysis. Br J Sports Med. 46, 927-930 doi:10.1136/bjsports-2011-085662.

109 Wilmot, E. G., Edwardson, C. L., Achana, F. A., Davies, M. J., Gorely, T., Gray, L. J., ... Biddle, J. H. (2012). Sedentary time in adults and the association with diabetes, cardiovascular disease and death: systematic review and meta-analysis. Diabetologia. 55(11), 2895-2905.

110 Latouche, C., Jowett, J. B., Carey, A. L., Bertovic, D. A, Owen, N., Dunstan, D. W., & Kingwell, B. A. (2013). Effects of breaking up prolonged sitting on skeletal muscle gene expression. J Appl Physiol (1985). 114(4), 453-60. doi: 10.1152/japplphysiol.00978.2012.

111 Wilmot, E. G., Edwardson, C. L., Achana, F. A., Davies, M. J., Gorely, T., Gray, L. J., ... Biddle, J. H. (2012). Sedentary time in adults and the association with diabetes, cardiovascular disease and death: systematic review and meta-analysis. Diabetologia. 55(11), 2895-2905.

- **Abnormal expression of genes involved with cardiovascular health:** Just five hours of uninterrupted sitting dramatically impacts the expression of genes involved with cellular growth and development, and many of these genetic changes are linked with cardiovascular disease.[112]

- **Disrupted appetite regulation and calorie overconsumption:** Even a single day of sitting for several hours disrupts the body's normal ability to regulate appetite (calorie intake) in accordance with biological need (i.e. calorie expenditure), and leads to a state of physiology that predisposes to calorie overconsumption, and thus, fat gain.[113] [114] [115] [116]

- **Insulin resistance:** Sitting induces profound levels of insulin resistance and predisposes to type II diabetes. One single day of sitting can significantly impact insulin sensitivity, and even when calorie intake is intentionally reduced to match the decreased level of activity, we still see insulin resistance.[117]

- **Fatigue:** Sitting and inactivity can lead to decreased number and health of mitochondria—the cellular energy generators—and thus slow down the metabolism over time.[118] [119] Less mitochondria tends to decrease physical

112 http://jap.physiology.org/content/114/4/453

113 http://www.ncbi.nlm.nih.gov/pubmed/22462636

114 http://www.ncbi.nlm.nih.gov/pubmed/14692601

115 http://www.dailymail.co.uk/health/article-1061462/Why-sitting-best-way-work-appetite.html

116 http://www.ncbi.nlm.nih.gov/pubmed/19752112

117 http://www.ncbi.nlm.nih.gov/pubmed/21067784

118 Timmons JA, Norrbom J, Schéele C, Thonberg H, Wahlestedt C, Tesch P.Expression profiling following local muscle inactivity in humans provides new perspective on diabetes-related genes. Genomics. 2006 Jan;87(1):165-72. Epub 2005 Dec 2.

119 Ringholm S, Biensø RS, Kiilerich K, Guadalupe-Grau A, Aachmann-Andersen NJ, Saltin B, Plomgaard P, Lundby C, Wojtaszewski JF,Calbet

energy levels over time, and predisposes to chronic fatigue.[120] (If you work a desk job and you're tired all the time, you should have a light bulb going off in your head right now).

- **Metabolism slowdown:** Even just a few hours of sitting induces startling levels of insulin resistance—the cell's ability to take in and utilize fuel.[121] It causes sugars and fats to sludge up in the blood, because they're not getting into the cell efficiently. The metabolism is cellular energy production. If energy isn't getting into the cell, the cell cannot produce energy. In other words sitting = metabolism slowdown. (Metabolism slowdown generally results in fatigue, various hormonal problems, and a predisposition to easy fat storage).

- **Dramatically decreased fat burning:** An enzyme called lipoprotein lipase (LPL) is the rate-limiting enzyme for the breakdown of fats circulating in the blood, and uptake of those fatty acids into muscle cells where they can be used as energy—or, to put it more simply, it helps you burn fat.[122] LPL activity is largely dependent on muscles being activated. If you're sitting still, LPL activity goes down dramatically. Muscle LPL activity is a prerequisite for the uptake and burning of fat that has been released from body fat stores.[123] To put it simply, sitting deactivates muscles,

JA, Pilegaard H. Bed rest reduces metabolic protein content and abolishes exercise-induced mRNA responses in human skeletal muscle. Am J Physiol Endocrinol Metab. 2011 Oct;301(4):E649-58. doi: 10.1152/ajpendo.00230.2011. Epub 2011 Jul 12.

120 http://www.sciencedaily.com/releases/2008/02/080228112008.htm

121 http://www.ncbi.nlm.nih.gov/pmc/articles/PMC3329818/#B24

122 Hamilton MT, Hamilton DG, Zderic TW. Role of low energy expenditure and sitting in obesity, metabolic syndrome, type 2 diabetes, and cardiovascular disease. Diabetes. Nov 2007;56(11):2655-2667.

123 Bey L, Hamilton MT. Suppression of skeletal muscle lipoprotein lipase activity during physical inactivity: a molecular reason to maintain daily low-intensity activity. The Journal of physiology. Sep 1 2003;551(Pt 2):673-682.

which in turn deactivates muscle LPL and brings fat burning to a grinding halt.

Perhaps the most significant thing to be aware of here, for anyone who works a desk job, is that sitting is an independent health risk factor—meaning that even if you do exercise, sitting for eight hours each day will *still* damage your health. [124] According to Thomas Yates, MD, "Even for people who are otherwise active, sitting for long stretches seems to be an independent risk factor for conditions like diabetes, cardiovascular disease, and kidney disease." [125] In other words, it's not just that people who sit a lot have worse health due to lack of exercise, it's that sitting by itself (regardless of how much exercise you do) causes harm. **Even if you work out at the gym four or five times a week for an hour, you will not undo the damage you're doing to your body through eight or twelve hours of sitting on your butt each day.**

As you can see, your movement behaviors throughout the day as you live your life are an unbelievably massive factor in your health, vitality, lifespan and body composition. To give you an idea of just how huge of a factor this is when it comes to body composition, take a look at the following data:[126]

---

124 Bauman A, Allman-Farinelli M, Huxley R, James WP. Leisure-time physical activity alone may not be a sufficient public health approach to prevent obesity–a focus on China. Obesity reviews : an official journal of the International Association for the Study of Obesity. Mar 2008;9 Suppl 1:119-126.

125 Wilmot, E. G., Edwardson, C. L., Achana, F. A., Davies, M. J., Gorely, T., Gray, L. J., ... Biddle, J. H. (2012). Sedentary time in adults and the association with diabetes, cardiovascular disease and death: systematic review and meta-analysis. Diabetologia. 55(11), 2895-2905.

126 http://www.nature.com/ejcn/journal/v59/n5/full/1602134a.html

OCCUPATION TYPE	NEAT
Chairbound	300
Seated work, no option of moving	700
Seated work: discretion and requirement to move	1,000
Standing work. E.g. homemaker, shop assistant	1,400
Strenuous work. E.g. agriculture	2,300

As you can see from this data, as we leave our jobs of tending to flocks and cultivating the fields and enter the cubicle, we are losing a whopping 1,000-1,500 calories per day. The amount of calories burned through a few hour-long workouts at the gym each week (roughly 150-400 calories burned per day on average) pales in comparison to the 1,000 plus calories extra each day that can be burned through a NEAT-optimized lifestyle.

One thing is abundantly clear from the latest research: NEAT is an absolutely massive factor when it comes to metabolic health and a lean body. According to Levine, "In the past fifty years—a blink of an eye in the history of all humankind—we got so good at developing ingenious time- and labor-saving devices that we literally started running the world not from our behinds. Our finely tuned human machine—the product of millions of years of evolution—is now short-circuiting as we've become completely glued to our chairs during the past twenty years. Today, our bodies are breaking down from obesity, high blood pressure, diabetes, cancer, depression, and the cascade of health ills and everyday malaise that come from what scientists such as myself named sitting disease."[127]

---

127 Levine, J. (2009). Move a Little, Lose a Lot. Crown Archetype.

A Summary of the Cellular/Hormonal Causes of Increased Body Fat Set-Point

There are five main cellular/hormonal causes of increased body fat set-point:

1. **Metabolically toxic foods** — Trans-fats, excess omega-6 PUFAs (poor omega 6:3 ratio), gluten (for those sensitive to it), foods containing hormone-altering chemical residues, and allergenic foods are the major culprits here.

2. **Chronic calorie overconsumption** — Even more important than any specific metabolically toxic foods is the metabolic toxicity of chronic calorie overconsumption itself that damages the cells' ability to take in and process nutrients. This is driven by a combination of a processed food diet, with appetite regulation disrupting factors like abnormal circadian rhythm and too much sitting/movement deficiency.

3. **Forced calorie deprivation (from diet and exercise)** — As I've explained in detail in earlier sections of this book, forcibly depriving the body of the calories it needs to function in an attempt to get fat loss is a horribly misguided and counterproductive strategy that eventually results in metabolism slowdown.

4. **Macronutrient and micronutrient deficiency** — Low-carb and low-fat fad diets can promote macronutrient deficiencies, which can result in hormonal problems and metabolism slowdown. Micronutrient deficiency from consuming a typical Western processed-food laden diet can result in the same metabolism slowing effect.

5. **Movement deficiency/excessive sitting** — Sitting down for hours and hours each day for years or decades is a killer. Not only will doing this completely sabotage your fat loss efforts—even if your nutrition and exercise habits are dialed in—but it will also worsen your cellular

health, bring your metabolism to a screeching halt, and dramatically shorten your lifespan.

Here is a nice little summary chart that gives you the visual for all of the neurological and cellular/hormonal factors I just explained:

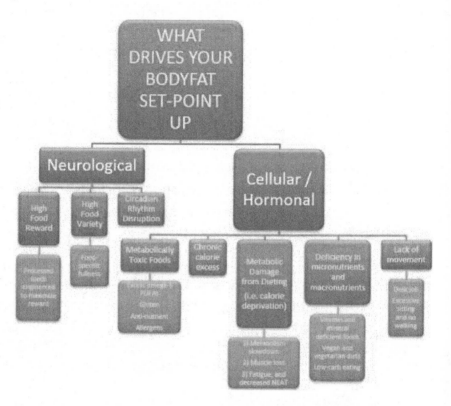

If you combine all of these cellular/hormonal and neurological factors that override the body fat set-point system, you have a super-potent recipe for massive amounts of fat gain.

Let me show you what I mean. Let's imagine a scenario that might look like what most of us living in the modern industrialized world typically experience:

What if we take a young girl at the age of 15, and:

- Give her access to endless variety of unnaturally rewarding processed foods that drive chronic overconsumption of calories.

- Disrupt her circadian rhythm with unnatural light exposure patterns on a daily basis, so her metabolism slows down, and her ability to regulate her calorie intake with biological need is disrupted.

- Put her on a diet of micronutrient deficient foods, which slow her metabolism.

- Give her a diet with ample metabolically toxic foods (like trans-fats, fried foods, hormone-altering chemical residues, and lots of vegetable oils) that further slow her metabolism.

- Have her sit down at a desk all day and rarely move her body, every day, for the next couple decades—bringing her metabolism to a grinding halt, shutting down the ability of her cells to burn fat, and further disrupting her ability to regulate appetite in accordance with her biological need.

- Then, when she gets a little fatter—as a result of all that metabolism slowdown, neurologically-driven calorie overconsumption, and appetite dysregulation—**tell her that the way to lose the fat is just to forcibly restrict her calorie intake (i.e. go on a diet)**, which will further starve her cells of energy, further slow the metabolism, and predispose to future fat gain.

Can you see how this situation that most of us are now in is the perfect storm for creating an obesity epidemic?

So, do you still think fat gain is just caused by "eating too many calories," and that fat loss is as simple as "eating fewer calories?"

Obviously, understanding fat gain and fat loss in the way I just presented to you is infinitely more sophisticated and scientifically complete than simply saying that fat gain and fat loss are a matter of your conscious decisions around how many calories you eat and how many times you go to the gym each week.

This paradigm allows us to address the real factors driving fat gain, instead of endlessly spinning our wheels with more restrictive diets and exercise programs that don't really get at the true underlying causes of why we got fat in the first place. It allows us to get fat loss by working with our biology instead of foolishly fighting against it.

The Blueprint to Eliminate All the Causes of Increased Body Fat Set-Point

Now that we understand that lasting fat loss is all about re-engaging the body fat set-point system by removing the factors from the modern environment that cause it to dysfunction, and we've already identified what those specific factors are, what we need to do now is simply *remove* those factors from our environment. This causes you to re-engage your body fat set-point system, driving your body fat set-point down effortlessly. Removing these environmental factors causes fat loss without any forced calorie restriction or suffering through hunger, and without any compensatory metabolic slowdown.

Just as all of the neurological and cellular/hormonal factors that disrupt the body fat set-point system all combine to create a state of physiology that drives *effortless fat gain* (i.e. puts you into a state where you will be chronically taking in more calories than you burn), if you address *all* of these factors, you can create a state of physiology that does precisely the opposite—it puts you into a state where fat burning exceeds fat storage, and as a result, drives effortless fat loss.

A hugely important point to be aware of: Not every person's fat gain is driven by the same factors. In fact, in my experience **there are two completely different kinds of overweight people:**

- First, there are the classic obese sedentary junk food eaters, and these people are overweight primarily due to a high food reward diet driving chronic calorie overconsumption. These people would benefit tremendously from a lower reward diet and getting back into harmony with their body's biological need for fuel. <u>In these people, the neurological causes of fat gain are dominant over the cellular/hormonal causes.</u> (Not to minimize the cellular and hormonal issues in many of these people, but they are typically secondary to the neurological causes of fat gain.)
- Then there are the chronic calorie counters, fad dieters, and exercise addicts. These are really a whole different breed of overweight people. They are often 10-30 pounds overweight while chronically trying to restrict calorie and carbohydrate intake. In other words, they are overweight despite following all the typical fat loss recommendations out there to restrict calories and eat low-carb and do tons of exercise. In reality, **they are overweight *as a result of following those recommendations***. That is, they've lowered their metabolic rate from chronic attempts at calorie restriction and fad diets, and their metabolisms have become so dysfunctional that they put on fat extremely easily, even with lots of exercise and minimal calorie intake. For these people, the cellular/hormonal causes of fat gain are much more significant than any issues of a high reward diet.

If you're a chronic dieter and exercise addict with a dysfunctional and disordered relationship with food, the solution for you is *not* more strict rules around your eating habits. You need to supply your body with the nutrients it needs to *repair* your broken metabolism and work on repairing your relationship with food (the books *Intuitive Eating* and Matt Stone's *Diet Recovery 2* are good places to start), not go on another restrictive diet. If that's the case for you, I suggest focusing on circadian rhythm and movement habits as you work on repairing your relationship with food. On the other hand, if you're a sedentary person eating tons of processed food, lowering the reward value of your diet and your overall calorie intake (not forcibly, but by eating whole foods) will be *extremely helpful.*

In other words, different combinations of all the neurological and cellular/hormonal factors can drive fat gain (and prevent fat loss) in different people. It's critical to be aware of that, and to tailor the solutions I'm about to present to *your* specific needs. For some people, they may already have their nutrition and exercise habits dialed in perfectly, but they work a desk job where they sit 12 hours a day and stare at a computer screen until midnight every night. **That disrupted circadian rhythm and movement deficiency can often completely sabotage everything they're doing with their diet and exercise program.** For someone else, it may be a diet packed with micronutrient-deficient foods that's holding them back. For someone else, they may be overweight due to being a cardio addict combined with a chronic calorie restrictor and low-carber for a decade, and now their metabolism has slowed down to a sloth's pace. For another person, it may be largely due to disrupted circadian rhythm from working night shifts or staying up late every night to watch TV. For another person, it may be their two decades of protein-deficient vegetarian eating that did it. For another person, it may have initially been processed foods that caused the initial fat gain, but now, as a result of doing years of low-carb dieting and exhausting cardio workouts they've caused themselves a bunch of metabolic damage that's keeping them fat. For another person, it may be that they have basically *everything* backwards—they're eating a diet full of micronutrient-deficient and highly rewarding processed foods, a diet rich with metabolic toxins, they have a chronically disrupted circadian rhythm, they've caused themselves lots of metabolic damage from years of chronic cardio workouts, and countless attempts at low calorie and low-carb weight loss diets, and on top of all that, they sit 12 hours a day.

Context is critical here, so please be cognizant of whether your issues are being driven by mostly neurological or cellular/hormonal causes, or both, and keep that in mind as you read through how to correct the sources of fat gain. Figure out which of these factors are most relevant to *you*.

So let's get into it and see exactly how to fix each one of the factors that drive up the body fat set-point. We'll start with the neurological factors.

The Blueprint to Eliminate the Neurological Causes of Fat Gain

The Neurological causes of obesity are highly rewarding foods, high food variety, and disrupted circadian rhythm. Here's how to correct each of those issues:

1. The High Food Reward Fix: If it doesn't run, fly, swim, or grow out of the ground, don't eat it! Eat only whole, unprocessed foods.

This step is critical to lowering the reward threshold in the brain and normalizing the brain's sensitivity to the reward value of food. What is that going to accomplish? It will allow you to get back into harmony with eating because of biological need, not because you're trying to give yourself pleasure. **Simply put, this step is the foundation of lasting fat loss.**

However, it is important to realize that the process of minimizing/eliminating highly rewarding processed food from your diet is an extremely individual thing, and there is no appropriate one-size-fits-all recommendation. Some people find it easiest if they include these foods occasionally in moderation and don't deal well with being "prohibited" from eating them (they might binge in response to an unsustainable level of constant restriction). For other people, if they allow themselves to have these foods occasionally they have difficulty stopping, and they may go on a week or two-week long junk food binge and completely wreck all their progress. For some people, it is helpful to have an initial period of complete abstinence from these foods, and many people then notice that their cravings for them eventually subside. For others, they work better with systematic moderation while still allowing themselves to indulge occasionally. But again, this is a very individual thing, and you have to choose the approach that works for your personality. Once you have successfully minimized or eliminated highly rewarding processed food from your diet for a period of at least a month, if you need to indulge once in a while because you're out to dinner with family or friends, or you just can't live without (insert specific highly rewarding processed food here), it's not a big deal. You don't need to be overly OCD or neurotic about this and start guilt-tripping yourself for eating so and so "forbidden food." Don't be so strict that you give yourself a disordered relationship with food. **Try to have a sustained period of either minimization or elimination of these foods first and get used to a whole food diet. Once you've done that and are completely comfortable eating a near-100% whole food diet, little indulgences every once in a while aren't a huge issue.**

Above all, train yourself to look at food at sustenance for your cells, *not* as a source of daily entertainment and pleasure. Eating for entertainment and pleasure is perfectly fine *occasionally*, but it causes big problems when done at every meal.

Eating whole unprocessed foods is *not* about depriving yourself of *tasty* food—it's not about avoiding things that taste good, like sweet foods or fatty foods. This is about depriving yourself of unnaturally neurologically rewarding food—food that has been professionally engineered to maximize the reward factor. That's it. You can eat the tastes you crave, just not in processed form.

In addition, whole natural food, unlike many processed foods, has a satiety to calorie ratio that is congruent with your body fat set-point system. That is, processed food overrides the body fat set-point system because it allows you to consume a lot more calories before actually feeling full—that means that processed food is fundamentally not in harmony with your biology. Processed foods frequently lead to passive calorie overconsumption simply due to the the extreme calorie density of those foods. Natural food allows the amount of fullness you feel while eating to be completely in tune with how many calories you actually ate. That is a critical factor to long-term fat loss success.

This strategy alone—eating only whole unprocessed foods—has been shown in the research to significantly drive down calorie intake and cause a tremendous amount of fat loss *without* any conscious effort to take in fewer calories and without *hunger*.[128] [129] Remember that the single biggest predictor of successful lasting weight loss is *hunger*.[130] In turn, modifying the food reward value of your diet is likely to be the single most powerful way to influence your hunger level.

Thus, losing fat without hunger is the mark of a strategy that is not just starving the body into fat loss but is actually lowering the body's set-point.

OVERCOME FOOD ADDICTION BY GIVING IN TO YOUR CRAVINGS. When you crave sweet things, eat sweet things. When you crave fatty things, eat fatty things. But—and that's a very big "but"—always choose **a whole, natural, and unprocessed food** to fulfill that craving. So when you crave sweet things, go to town on fruit. When you crave salty things like French fries, cut up some sweet potatoes or potatoes, rub them with some coconut oil, put a bunch of salt all over them, and stick 'em in the oven. By doing this, you've just made yourself

---

128 Ryberg, M., Sandberg, S., Mellberg, C., Stegle, O., Lindahl, B., Larsson, C., … Olsson, T. (2013). A Palaeolithic-type diet causes strong tissue-specific effects on ectopic fat deposition in obese postmenopausal women. J Int Med. 274 (1), 67–76. doi: 10.1111/joim.12048

129 Lindeberg, S., Jönsson, T., Granfeldt, Y., Borgstrand, E., Soffman, J., Sjöström, K., & Ahrén, B. (2007). A Palaeolithic diet improves glucose tolerance more than a Mediterranean-like diet in individuals with ischaemic heart disease. Diabetologia. 50(9), 1795-807.

130
http://www.ncbi.nlm.nih.gov/pubmed/23512619?dopt=Abstract&holding=npg

whole food French fries that are infinitely more nutritious, without being fried in metabolically toxic polyunsaturated fats. If you crave fatty foods, have some raw cheese. If you crave sweet and fatty foods together, have some grass-fed yogurt with coconut cream and berries. There's no excuse here. I'm not asking you to deprive yourself of the calories you need or of the taste you crave, only of processed food. This strategy will minimize (and likely eliminate) any psychological suffering associated with fat loss eating, because it still allows you to eat the quantity and tastes you crave. No forced deprivation from calories or tastes means effortless fat loss. One caveat: You do have to break your addiction-like habits with processed foods before being able to really trust your cravings. Once you have broken the addiction, learn to see your cravings as intelligent signals from your body telling you what it needs. And then feed it the most nutrient-dense whole food version of the stuff it craves.

If you're currently eating a diet full of processed foods, making the effort to transition to a whole-foods diet is almost guaranteed to be life transforming.

2. The High Food Variety Fix: Eliminate calorie overconsumption by eating simple meals.

By eating simple meals with just a few whole foods, you have a massively powerful strategy for fat loss. This is one of Guyenet's fundamental strategies for lowering body fat set-point.[131] Just as we know that high variety of foods drives up total calorie intake, we also know that lowering food variety (eating simple meals) is an incredibly powerful strategy that can cause massive amounts of fat loss that lasts. Again, this is such a simple concept that people have a tendency to overlook it, but if you actually apply it, it's incredibly powerful. Like I said, just this one strategy—even if you don't do any of the other things that I've

---

131 Guyenet, S. (2012, August 29). Obesity; Old solutions for a new problem. 2011 Ancestral Health Symposium UCLA. Retrieved from https://www.youtube.com/watch?v=srqFz0fO8xk.

discussed in this book—will cause massive fat loss, and there is good scientific research to back that up.[132]

Eating simple meals doesn't mean you have to eat only one food (like a meal of just a couple of potatoes and nothing else, or a steak and nothing else). I'm talking about limiting your meals to a few foods (perhaps one animal food, plus a fruit and/or vegetable) in each meal and to prepare those foods simply—to not be excessively gourmet and elaborate with fancy sauces and flavorings.

By arranging these whole natural foods in simple meals with just a few components, you are eliminating the possibility of food-specific fullness working against you and causing you to over-consume calories beyond your body's biological need.

This doesn't need to be about depriving yourself of anything that tastes good, or eating nothing but potatoes, or nothing but salads, or nothing but cheese. You can still have variety in your diet and eat things that taste good. Just use whole foods and keep your individual meals simple. Note that this applies more to the first type of overweight person—the person on the processed food diet—rather than the person who's already been doing too much dietary restriction.

3. The Circadian Rhythm Fix: Reset circadian rhythm.

To reset your body's circadian rhythm, you're going to combine a protocol of ample light (of the right spectrum) during the daytime, supplement with specific micronutrients, and minimize blue light exposure after sunset. This simple combination is an incredibly powerful way to restore normal, healthy circadian rhythms and eliminate sleep troubles forever.

For millions of years (up until the last century or so), human activity paralleled the rise and fall of the sun. In the modern world, however, we spend most of our days indoors under artificial lights, and for many hours at night. When we should be

---

132 Cabanac, M., & Rabe, E. F. (1976). Influence of a monotonous food on body weight regulation in humans. Physiol Behav. 17(4), 675-8.

in either darkness or in firelight (mostly red light wavelengths), we now have tons of blue light entering our eyes from all of our televisions, smart phones, and computers. As a result, we have become out of sync with the sun, and many of us have chronic sleep and hormonal problems.

The fix is very simple:

1. Get lots of light during the day.
2. Eliminate light after sunset, or at least light in the blue spectrum.
3. Supplement with micronutrients that most of us are deficient in like magnesium which is linked to poor sleep.

The main part of this fix is pretty simple: More light during the day, and less light at night.

It's a pretty simple concept to understand, but many people in the modern world have terrible difficulty putting it into practice.

You must get light—real sunlight ideally, or if that's not possible, a full spectrum artificial light source—during the daytime every single day. Generally speaking, the more the better, but at a minimum, 1-2 hours each day of either sunlight or a light therapy box. The best low-priced device currently on the market for this purpose can be found on <u>my recommended products</u> page under "Circadian Rhythm Reset." There are other higher-priced devices you can find on Amazon which work great as well if you fancy a different look.

If you're not getting outdoors and getting natural sunlight, you should use this device in the morning after you wake up for 30 minutes (you can use it while getting ready in front of the mirror, meditating, cooking breakfast, working at your computer, etc.). That's enough to provide you with tons of benefits and reset circadian rhythm, but if you want to amplify the effect, you can also use it for 10-20 minutes every few hours as you're sitting at your desk working throughout the day. Intense light exposure from wake-up until noon is strongly linked with having a leaner body.[133]

Eliminate blue light after sunset:

Just as important as getting ample light during the daytime to suppress melatonin is eliminating light in the blue spectrum after sunset to make sure melatonin is *not* suppressed after it's dark outside. You want to have the absence of artificial light from room lighting, computer screens, cell phone screens, and TVs after sunset. At the very least, avoid blue spectrum light in the evening, since it's the blue spectrum that's responsible for melatonin suppression.

How can you eliminate the blue spectrum only? You have a couple of choices. One is to install free f.lux software (http://justgetflux.com/) on your computer and smart phone, and this will almost completely eliminate the blue spectrum of light on the screens of those devices. Alternatively, you can use blue light blocking screens on your computer and phone, which actually block blue light even more effectively than f.lux, and they work for your TV as well, which f.lux doesn't. (Note: If you have severe sleep troubles, and you're serious about fixing the problem, you should use the blue-blocking screens rather than f.lux, as they block blue light more completely.)

For computer screens and TVs:
https://www.lowbluelights.com/products.asp?cid=55
For phones:
https://www.lowbluelights.com/products.asp?cid=57
You may also get blue-blocking sunglasses (see the recommended products page on my website: http://www.ariwhitten.com/recommended-products), which will effectively eliminate all light in the blue spectrum from entering your eyes from room lighting as well as electronic screens, though it does require that you wear goofy sunglasses

---

133 Morning rays keep off the pounds. Retrieved from:
    http://www.northwestern.edu/newscenter/stories/2014/04/morning-rays-keep-off-the-pounds.html

around your house at night. If you prefer not to do that, then you want to get the blue-blocking screens for your phone, computer, and TV if you plan on using those devices after sunset.

While avoiding TV in general is best, if you absolutely cannot live without watching TV before bed, you can *still* do it without disrupting your circadian rhythm by simply using one of the blue light blocking screens over your TV.

If you do not either get the blue-blocking screen for your TV or want to wear the amber sunglasses in your house, then you'll have to avoid watching TV within 2-3 hours of bedtime.

So there's really no excuse. Even if you absolutely must use your cellphone, computer, and TV incessantly after sunset, you can eliminate all blue light emanating from them by using either f.lux, blue-blocking glasses, or by using blue-blocking screens.

By doing this, you allow your brain to produce melatonin at the time when it's supposed to and you keep your circadian rhythm intact.

Optional: You may use light in the yellow, orange, and red spectrum in the evening as a source of indoor light.

Perhaps coincidently, or more likely by evolutionary design since humans evolved in the glow of firelight, the yellow, orange, and red wavelengths don't suppress melatonin production the way white and blue wavelengths do.[134] [135] [136] [137]

---

134 Burkhart, K. & Phelps, J. R. (2009). Amber lenses to block blue light and improve sleep: a randomized trial. Chronobiol Int. 26(8), 1602-12. doi: 10.3109/07420520903523719.

135 Cajochen, C., Münch, M., Kobialka, S., Kräuchi, K., Steiner, R., Oelhafen, P., … Wirz-Justice, A. (2005). High sensitivity of human melatonin, alertness, thermoregulation, and heart rate to short wavelength light. The Journal of Clinical Endocrinology & Metabolism. 90(3). http://dx.doi.org/10.1210/jc.2004-0957 .

136 Figueiro, M. G., Bierman, A., Plitnick, B. & Rea, M. S. (2009). Preliminary evidence that both blue and red light can induce alertness at night. BMC Neurosci. 10, 105. doi: 10.1186/1471-2202-10-105.

137 Kayumov, L., Casper, R. F., Hawa, R. J., Perelman, B., Chung, S. A., Sokalsky, S. & Shapiro, C. M. (2005). Blocking low-wavelength light prevents nocturnal melatonin suppression with no adverse effect on performance

Another option, rather than using software and blue-blocking glasses, is to shift to a low-wattage bulb with yellow, orange, or red light in your house after the sun goes down. The bulbs on my recommended products page are examples, but really any red-colored or orange-colored bulb will work.

In addition, fire and candlelight are wonderful options for lighting your home at night without suppressing melatonin. If you're unwilling to do this, at least try to dim the lights after sunset and minimize light exposure, along with using f.lux or blue-blocking screens on your electronic devices.

If you get in the habit of using amber/red bulbs and/or candles, you may find that you actually like it and that it adds a wonderful ambience to your home.

Sleep in complete darkness:

In addition to ample light exposure during the day and minimal blue light exposure while you're awake in the evening, you want to sleep in complete darkness. Do this by unplugging anything emitting light (alarm clocks, nightlights, etc), and either use blackout shades on all windows, or wear an eye mask. I recommend the blackout shades, as the eye mask can sometimes disturb sleep. Sleeping in complete darkness is a powerful way to ensure deeper sleep. In surveys of people who struggle sleeping, room darkness is consistently ranked as being critical to a good night's sleep.[138]

Correct your micronutrient deficiencies:

Magnesium:

Remember, most people are magnesium-deficient and would benefit from dramatically increasing their magnesium intake. Oranges, cacao (dark chocolate), and coffee are great sources of

---

during simulated shift work. The Journal of Clinical Endocrinology & Metabolism. 90(5). doi: http://dx.doi.org/10.1210/jc.2004-2062.

138 Breus, M. (2012, April 29). How Sleep-Friendly Is Your Bedroom? Retrieved from http://www.huffingtonpost.com/dr-michael-j-breus/sleep-bedroom_b_1455850.html

magnesium that can be consumed daily. Additionally, for those with poor sleep or who are chronically fatigued, I recommend supplementing with oral magnesium citrate or glycinate just before bed (1/2-1tsp). Transdermal magnesium is actually the fastest way to correct magnesium deficiency (much more efficient than oral magnesium), and by spraying magnesium oil on your body liberally each day and/or taking magnesium-rich Epsom salt baths regularly before bed (whichever is more convenient for you), you are likely to notice profound effects on your sleep quality very quickly. If you use magnesium oil, you can spray your body at any time of the day, but you want to make sure to also do it right before bed. You can either rinse off in the shower (after at least 20 minutes of having the magnesium on your body), or simply leave it on if it doesn't bother you. Magnesium is a very powerful tool that you will notice instant effects from, and for many people, magnesium alone has cured their insomnia. Magnesium citrate/glycinate (the oral forms), magnesium oil (which is magnesium salt mixed with water for topical application), and Epsom salt can all be found on Amazon or in your local supplement store. (See my recommended products page if you want my recommended brands).

If you follow the above steps, you have the blueprint for eliminating all of the neurological causes of fat gain. This is the first and most important prerequisite to lasting fat loss. If you don't eliminate these neurological causes of obesity, you will struggle trying to lose fat (and more than likely you'll fail) over and over again for the rest of your life. If you do the above fixes for food reward, food variety, and the circadian rhythm, you may just find the fat effortlessly coming off.

But since we want an absolutely complete system to correct every possible factor that contributes to fat gain, let's take it a step further and correct all the cellular/hormonal factors that drive up the body fat set-point, as well.

The Blueprint to Eliminate the Cellular/Hormonal Causes of Fat Gain

In terms of cellular and hormonal causes of fat gain, we have metabolic damage from chronic calorie overconsumption, metabolic damage from metabolically toxic foods, metabolic damage from forced calorie deprivation, and deficiencies in either macronutrients or micronutrients. Let's get into how to fix each one of these issues:

1. The Fix for the Metabolic Toxicity of Chronic Calorie Overconsumption: Focus on eating whole unprocessed foods, with a high protein intake.

The fix here is fairly straightforward: The metabolic damage from a chronic excess of calories is largely already fixed by following the principles in the section above for eliminating the neurological causes of increased body fat set-point. By fixing your circadian rhythm and eating simple meals of only whole, unprocessed foods, you will stop the chronic overconsumption of calories. In addition, **I highly recommend putting a focus on <u>eating at least 1g of protein per pound of lean body mass each day.</u>** (Use this calculator to determine your lean body mass: <u>CLICK HERE</u>. If you don't know your body fat percentage, just aim for close to 1g of protein per pound of bodyweight each day). **This should be your daily goal.** As previously stated, **high protein intake and a whole-foods diet are incredibly powerful strategies for fat loss**—particularly when you combine them with all the other strategies I'm presenting to you in this book.

2. The Metabolically Toxic Foods Fix: Minimize/eliminate metabolically toxic foods from your diet.

As noted earlier in the book, there are several types of foods which are potentially metabolically toxic foods for some people: Gluten (for those who are gluten-sensitive), vegetable oils (more than likely), trans-fats, allergens, foods containing hormone-altering chemical residues, and improperly prepared grains, legumes, lentils, nuts and seeds (only if you consume them as a very large portion of your diet).

As far as the metabolically toxic foods like trans-fats (fried foods, and packaged foods with hydrogenated vegetable oils) and allergens, the fix is simple: **Get them completely out of your diet.**

If you wish to consume large amounts of grains, legumes, nuts, and seeds, it's smart to eat properly prepared versions of these foods that have been soaked/sprouted and/or cooked, where appropriate.

But again, my intention here is not to be just another diet book that gives you a long list of forbidden foods. So I am very intentionally keeping discussion of various "bad foods" to a minimum so that people do not fixate on this factor. My philosophy is about figuring out what the best sources of nutrients are and eating those foods as the primary staples of your diet. Focus so much on eating the best sources of nutrients that you don't have room for anything but high quality foods.

3. The Fix for Metabolic Damage from Forced Calorie Restriction: Eat according to your biological need, don't be a cardio junkie, and do NOT forcibly restrict calories.

As I explained in the first half of this book, not only is forced calorie deprivation *not* an effective fat loss strategy, it is actually *counterproductive,* as for many people, it creates compensatory metabolic slowdown that often causes them to get fatter over time. It is for this reason that I do *not* ever recommend forced calorie restriction. You do technically need to be in a state where your body is burning more calories than you take in, in order to lose fat. However, this should be done *not* by forcibly trying to do this, but by creating the conditions (i.e. following the principles I am outlining here) that allow this process to occur naturally and effortlessly. In other words, doing it by working with your biology, rather than against it. As numerous studies have now demonstrated, by following the principles I've outlined (such as eating a whole foods diet with simple meals, fixing your circadian rhythm, improving micronutrient status, etc.), you can achieve massive fat loss effortlessly, without forced calorie restriction. That is really the holy grail of fat loss—effortless fat loss, and fat loss not by starving the body of calories, but by actually lowering the body's preferred level of fat mass (the set-point).

The fix here is pretty simple: Eat *according to your biological need.* That means:

- Do *not* try to forcibly restrict calories below what your body is telling you it needs—when you are hungry, eat.
- Eat when you're hungry and *only* when you're hungry—not out of boredom or to give yourself pleasure.
- Eat the amount your body is telling you that you need and *stop* eating when you're full.

Doing this prevents and repairs the metabolic damage that comes from forced calorie deprivation.

4. The Metabolic Damage From Fad Diets Fix: Reverse the metabolic damage from macronutrient-restricted fad diets by consuming nutrients you're deficient in.

If you've done any fad macronutrient restriction diets like veganism/vegetarianism or low-fat or low-carb eating (which all typically cause metabolic damage over time), eating the macronutrients that you've been deficient in (from whole food sources) will help undo the metabolic damage that comes from these diets. If you're overweight and you've been on a low-protein vegetarian diet for the last ten years, eating whole-food animal proteins (fish, shellfish, dairy, and eggs) is extremely therapeutic and can help correct the protein deficiency and micronutrient deficiencies common on vegetarian/vegan diets.[139] If you've been restricting fat, eating whole food fats like coconut and grass-fed butter is powerful medicine. And especially if you've been brainwashed by the low-carb fad into thinking that forcibly restricting your carbohydrate intake is "good for you," eating whole-food carbohydrates like oranges and sweet potatoes will provide you with a massive change in your energy level, physical and cognitive performance, and mood. (Remember, carbs are your friends). Don't fight your cravings—give your body what it needs.

5. The Micronutrient Deficiency Fix: Reverse the metabolic damage from micronutrient deficiency by eating an ultra micronutrient-rich whole foods diet.

Now, if you've been eating a processed food diet or the standard American diet, you've been eating a micronutrient-deficient diet. Most people are deficient in numerous micronutrients, and correcting these micronutrient deficiencies can have a significant impact on your body composition. A fascinating and important study that supports this idea was just published in the journal *Obesity*, and showed that, compared to a placebo, a low-dose multivitamin caused obese volunteers to lose 7 lbs. (3.2 kg) of fat mass in six months, mostly from the abdominal region. The supplement also reduced LDL (bad cholesterol) by 27%, increased HDL (good cholesterol) by a whopping 40%, and increased resting energy expenditure.[140]

---

139 Kresser, C. (2014). Why you should think twice about vegetarian and vegan diets. Retrieved from http://chriskresser.com/why-you-should-think-twice-about-vegetarian-and-vegan-diets

140 Li, Y., Wang, C., Zhu, K., Feng, R. N., & Sun, C. H. (2010). Effects of multivitamin and mineral supplementation on adiposity, energy

Guyenet had this to say on this study:

"Many nutrients act together to create health, and multiple insufficiencies may contribute to disease. This may be why single nutrient supplementation trials usually don't find much. Another possibility is that obesity can result from a number of different nutrient insufficiencies, and the cause is different in different people. This study may have seen a large effect because it corrected many different insufficiencies. This result, once again, kills the simplistic notion that body fat is determined exclusively by voluntary food consumption and exercise behaviors (sometimes called the 'calories in, calories out' idea, or 'gluttony and sloth'). In this case, a multivitamin was able to increase resting energy expenditure and cause fat loss without any voluntary changes in food intake or exercise, suggesting metabolic effects and a possible downward shift of the body fat 'set-point' due to improved nutrient status."[141]

What he is saying here supports my long-held suspicions that micronutrient deficiency can drive up the body fat set-point. With an ample supply of micronutrients in the diet, the body is less likely to overconsume calories, which leads to the accumulation of body fat. And if you're already overweight, correcting micronutrient deficiencies and supplying the cells with an abundant supply of the vitamins and minerals they need to produce energy will therefore lead to loss of body fat, just as it did in this study. How does it do this? You'll notice in that study found that the multivitamin increased "resting energy expenditure." That means it increased the amount of calories their bodies were burning at rest—while sitting at their desk at work, while lounging around at the house, and even while they were asleep. In other words, optimal micronutrient status speeds up your metabolism!

expenditure and lipid profiles in obese Chinese women. Int J Obes (Lond), 34(6), 1070-7. doi: 10.1038/ijo.2010.14

141 Guyenet, S. (2010). Low micronutrient intake may contribute to obesity. Retrieved from http://wholehealthsource.blogspot.com/2010/06/low-micronutrient-intake-may-contribute.html

As far as the practical implications of this multivitamin study, Guyenet offers some words of wisdom to those who might seek to continue eating their normal diet and just add in a multivitamin on top of it to correct any issues with their nutrition: "Does this mean we should all take multivitamins to stay or become thin? No. There is no multivitamin that can match the completeness and balance of a nutrient-dense, whole food, omnivorous diet." [142]

The solution is simple: Eat a super-micronutrient-rich whole food diet full of fruits and vegetables. Eating a whole food diet instantly doubles the micronutrient content of the diet. By eating whole natural foods and lots of fruits and vegetables, you can slowly flush the micronutrients back into your body and give your cells the nutrients they need to function and produce energy optimally (i.e. enhance metabolic rate), which is critical to enhancing your fat loss efforts.

6. The Sitting/Movement Deficiency Fix: Stand up and MOVE every single day!

Sitting and being sedentary is extremely damaging to your health, and working a desk job where you sit for hours and hours each day makes it virtually impossible to lose lots of fat—even if your nutrition and exercise habits are dialed in perfectly.

Fat gain is not being driven by a deficiency in P90X and Crossfit workouts, and thus trying to approach fat loss by going on an exercise program isn't likely to get you very far. Exercise is certainly part of a healthy lifestyle, but if your goal is fat loss, rather than concerning yourself with how much exercise you do or don't do, a far wiser thing to focus on is how much *sitting* you do or don't do. Simply put, sitting for a large portion of each day on a daily basis, year after year, is a great way to make yourself sick and fat, and completely sabotage all your efforts at fat loss using nutrition and exercise. Likewise, one of the most powerful

---

142 Guyenet, S. (2010). Low micronutrient intake may contribute to obesity. Retrieved from http://wholehealthsource.blogspot.com/2010/06/low-micronutrient-intake-may-contribute.html

strategies in existence that you can take to improve your health, your metabolism, and your body composition is to **minimize sitting during the day and move your body as constantly as possible.**

Notice I did not say just "work out" or "do more exercise." The act of sitting less and standing and moving more is far more important than worrying about doing workouts. Simple ultra-low intensity movement throughout the day can be way more powerful than even doing three or four intense hour-long workouts at the gym each week—*way* more powerful. Why? Simple. Because movement is a requirement for normal healthy cell function. The proper way to understand movement is not as some trivial supplementary sort of thing that you can do to enhance your health or lose some fat—<u>movement is as essential to healthy cell function as oxygen, water, and food</u>. And depriving your body of movement by sitting in a chair all day is the equivalent of starving your body of oxygen, water, and nutrients.

I believe that if we want to create the optimal movement blueprint for health and a lean body, we must first discover, and then follow, the movement and activity patterns that our species is designed for. We must, in other words, move in harmony with our genetic design. A recent study titled "Achieving Hunter-gatherer Fitness in the 21st Century: Back to the Future" has set the stage and made it easy for us to do exactly that. The group of scientists who did this study thoroughly analyzed the activity patterns of hunter-gatherer tribes and hominid fossil remains in order to establish a model of the ideal activity patterns for us to follow in order to express ideal health. I'll let the scientists themselves elaborate on this idea in their words: "The systematic displacement from a very physically active lifestyle in our natural outdoor environment to a sedentary, indoor lifestyle is at the root of many of the ubiquitous chronic diseases that are endemic in our culture. The intuitive solution is to simulate the indigenous human activity pattern to the extent that this is possible and practically achievable...with a **focus on realigning our daily physical activities with the archetype that is encoded within** our genome."[143] So then, what exactly are natural human activity patterns? Based on studying modern day hunter-gatherer tribes and anthropological evidence, these researchers determined the following principles of natural human activity patterns (note that the most important and relevant points are in bold):

CHARACTERISTICS OF A HUNTER-GATHERER FITNESS PROGRAM

- They did large amounts of walking every day. Our ancestors typically walked between 4 to 10 miles daily.
- After a very hard day of physical activity, they typically followed it by an easier day. They made sure to include ample time for rest and recuperation after hard work.
- They moved around on dirt or grass, not asphalt and cement.
- A few times a week, they did occasional bursts of very high intensity movements like sprinting, and these bursts were followed by adequate rest and recovery before another burst of exertion.
- They lifted, carried, dragged, pushed, chopped, and pulled heavy objects like stones or blocks of wood, regularly.
- They did all their exercise outdoors in the natural world.
- They often did physical activity in a social context in small bands of individuals out hunting or foraging.
- With the exception of only the very young and the extremely old, everyone did lots of physical activity, every day, for their entire lives.

The obvious implication from this is that these people spent most of their days standing up, walking, tending to the fields and the flocks, and otherwise *moving their bodies*—not sitting at a desk all day! And this isn't just a trivial fact of history—much research

---

143 Cordain, L., Lavie, C., O' Keefe, J., Vogel, R. (2010). Achieving Hunter-gatherer Fitness in the 21st Century: Back to the Future. The American Journal of Medicine, Vol 123, No 12, December 2010

in recent years has now made it clear that moving throughout the day is actually a *requirement* for normal cellular and metabolic function. In other words, if you sit all day, your metabolism can't work properly. If we want optimal health, vitality, a fast metabolism, and a lean body, we need to <u>move</u>.

Unfortunately, we now live in a world that requires many of us to be working at a computer most of the day. So how can we reconcile our body's needs for movement with our modern lifestyle of being in front of a computer all day?

Well, that's exactly what I'm about to show you. If you want to read a really in-depth and elaborate solution to accomplishing that in every aspect of your life, read Dr. James Levine's *Move a Little, Lose a Lot.* I like to keep things simple, so I'm going to take this absolutely massive factor that's critical to your health, lifespan, energy level, and body composition, and I'm going to give you an ultra-simple and ultra-powerful solution.

The ideal daily movement habits for fat loss and optimal health look like this:

1. Work standing up, and ideally, walking slowly.

During the day, <u>sit as little as possible</u>! Try to move your body almost constantly throughout the day. As Dr. Levine says, "there shouldn't be an hour of the day where you're sitting still."[144] You don't need to be doing exercise, just ultra-low intensity gentle movement. To give you an idea of how powerful this can be, take a look at the following graph.

---

144 BBC Documentary. The Truth About Exercise.

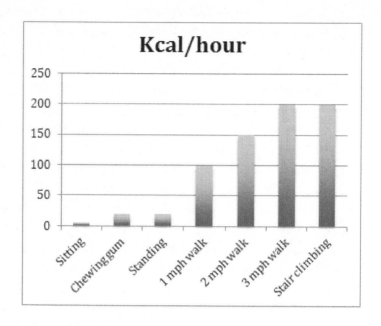

Kcal/hour

Sitting · Chewing gum · Standing · 1 mph walk · 2 mph walk · 3 mph walk · Stair climbing

Compare walking at an incredibly slow speed on a treadmill desk to just sitting at your desk like you normally would. Sitting is basically the same caloric expenditure as normal rest like sleeping—just 5% or so more calories burned than just basal metabolic rate (which is the amount of calories your body burns in a state of bed rest—just basic life functions, like breathing and keeping your heart beating). Now look at say, using a treadmill desk and walking at a very slow speed while you work all day—it elevates caloric expenditure by 125%-225% over basal metabolic rate. This is *huge*! Here is Levine's words on this data: "...watch what happens as the average volunteer goes from sitting still as a stone to standing to briskly walking. **The mere act of standing on your feet burns three times as many calories as sitting in your seat. Any little movement on top of that (even something as minute as chewing gum!) creates even greater metabolic spikes. When you walk, your metabolism literally blasts off**...it's easy to see how the loss of constant daily acitivty has decreased our natural calorie-burning metabolism by more than 50 percent."[145] In addition, irrespective of the amount of calories burned, the simple act of standing up dramatically ramps up activity of the fat burning enzyme LPL, which is critical to allowing fats to get out of the blood and into the muscles where they can be burned.[146]

Do this completely non-strenuous activity for several hours each day (which takes basically *zero* effort, and no extra time compared to your normal day) and you have a massively powerful way to transform your body that is essentially effortless. In fact, your body will actually feel *better* doing this compared to sitting, your posture will improve, you will likely be *more* productive, and you will actually feel *more* energetic! It doesn't get much better than that.

As Dr. James Levine notes in his book, <u>Move a Little, Lose a Lot</u>, many of his clients have transformed their bodies from these simple NEAT increasing strategies that require basically no time or effort—just a little bit of conscious habit creation initially, and then they are easily self-sustaining. If you want to learn more about this and see Dr. Levine talking about how damaging sitting is for our body, watch this documentary: <u>BBC's The Truth About Exercise.</u> **This fantastic documentary will drastically change the way you think about exercise and changing your body. If you're currently working a desk job, this information is life-transforming.** (Note: NEAT and sitting is discussed starting around the 32:00 mark, but you'd be smart to watch the whole thing, even if you think you know it all). It clearly shows that you can burn upwards of 500 or even 1,000 extra calories per day by changing your NEAT habits, which is *way* more significant than most exercise routines—and doesn't require a *drop* of sweat or really any significant exertion.

---

145 Levine, J. (2009). Move a Little, Lose a Lot. Crown Archetype.

146 Bey L, Hamilton MT. Suppression of skeletal muscle lipoprotein lipase activity during physical inactivity: a molecular reason to maintain daily low-intensity activity. The Journal of physiology. Sep 1 2003;551(Pt 2):673-682.

As to how you want to accomplish this, there are a few different options:

The absolute most powerful option is this: Get a treadmill desk and spend your day working at your computer *while* walking very slowly. As you saw from looking at the graph above, this is where the metabolism takes off and you get huge increases in calorie expenditure from NEAT each day, with really no effort. Even more important than the calories burned is the simple fact that this movement is allowing your cells and your metabolism to function the way they should be. Shifting to a treadmill desk requires a big change in habit, but not a big change in effort. It requires no real effort, and it actually feels rather good! Your posture improves, your energy level improves, and your productivity improves—all while you're radically increasing your metabolic health and putting your physiology in a state where fat loss becomes very easy. (Some people also use a portable mini stair stepper and do very gentle stepping while working at a standing desk, but for others, this may have too much up and down motion).

Less ideal, but still a good alternative is to get a standing desk. You can buy, make, or modify your current desk into a standing desk. Then spend your days standing 50-80% of the day, and never sitting for more than 45 minutes at a time without taking a break to stand up and move around. (The *GeekDesk* is electronically adjustable, so you can alternate between standing and sitting). Alternatively, you can get a cycling desk, or get a cheap portable under-desk cycle, and sit down at your cycling desk and pedal throughout the day as you work.

The least effective alternative (but still way better than sitting all day) is to sit as you would normally during the day, but set a timer to go off every 40-60 minutes throughout the day, and when it goes off, get up and move for 30-60 seconds—play on a wobble board, or balance on a balance disk, or use a little portable stair stepper, or balance on your hands and knees on a stability ball, for 30-60 seconds. Then go back to work.

Just interrupting the sitting for a minute or two with very gentle movement can have profound health benefits. Though you will not get some of the more profound metabolic benefits of working while on a treadmill desk or even the standing desk.

Again, by far the best choice here is a treadmill desk, which can either be bought in full (see my recommended products page on my website), or you can make your own setup using your regular desk and buying a cheap treadmill. The pre-made whole setup is rather expensive, so many people may wish to make their own setup using their existing desk.

If you just absolutely positively cannot use a treadmill desk, or it seems "ridiculous" or "weird" or "extreme" to you, just get a standing desk. This factor is too important to not be doing one of these two things. If you absolutely can't do even that, get a portable cycle to put under your desk. One way or another, make sure you're moving your body the majority of the day. Just one last time for emphasis: Make sure you're implementing this strategy. **Sitting all day is a great way to completely sabotage all your fat loss efforts through nutrition and exercise, and slowly wreck your metabolism. Stand up and *move!***

2. Go for at least one walk every day.

Once you have a foundation of not sitting so much and standing while working, if possible, start going for 1-2 walks each day, ideally outside enjoying nature and sunlight, if possible. These walks can be from fifteen minutes to one hour or more, depending on preference. Breathe. Meditate. Enjoy it. (Note: This is not really necessary if you're using a treadmill desk throughout the day. But do still make sure you get outdoors regularly).

3. Ramp up your daily NEAT—it can be incredibly powerful for fat loss. Move throughout the day!

If you work out at the gym, you might burn something like 300-400 calories per workout. Figure about 1,000-1,400 calories total for these three or four workouts each week. Divide that by the seven days of the week, and you get somewhere between 100-300 calories per day for most people. With strong NEAT habits, you can double or triple this easily. Moreover, the actual effect on enhancing insulin sensitivity, cellular health, hormonal health, and speeding up the metabolism will be *greater* in someone doing some simple NEAT-enhancing habits throughout the day than in someone who is mostly sedentary but does four or five gym workouts each week. Active couch potatoes (people with high NEAT but no gym workouts) are metabolically *healthier* than lazy exercisers (people who work desk jobs but do gym workouts).[147] Driving up your daily NEAT through walking, and fidgeting/playing throughout the day while working at your standing desk can burn huge amounts of calories (much more than most people's workout programs) and dramatically accelerate your fat loss results. Use it! It's extremely powerful. Obviously using a treadmill desk is the best way to do this, but if you're using one of the other options, there are some simple tweaks you can do that require minimal time and basically *zero* strain which can dramatically improve your metabolic function, your energy levels, your health, and your body:

- Stand up and pace while taking phone calls. Walk up stairs wherever you go rather than take the elevator.

- Answer texts and emails on your phone while on a portable stair stepper next to your desk.

- Hold walking meeting where you talk things over with colleagues while on the move.

- Buy a portable stepper and use it while reading or on phone calls.

- Here's a NEAT Little Trick (excuse the pun): If you are using a regular seated desk or standing (non-treadmill) desk, one very helpful little tool for training new NEAT-related habits is a free tool you can download on your

---

147 Matthews CE, Jurj AL, Shu XO, et al. Influence of exercise, walking, cycling, and overall nonexercise physical activity on mortality in Chinese women. American journal of epidemiology. Jun 15 2007;165(12):1343-1350

computer and/or phone: A Mindfulness bell. Use it to serve as a reminder to do NEAT movements. You can set the timer to go off every 30 minutes, and every time it goes off, do thirty seconds of stair stepping on a cheap portable stair stepper, or balance on the wobble board for a bit, or stretch, or play with a stress ball, dance a little, etc. E.g. Every 30 minutes when you hear the bell, do some stretches or flat-back posture exercises against a wall, do some gentle mobility exercises like these here: (http://bit.ly/1H0F1Bg), try to balance for a 30 seconds on a balance disc, etc. These are examples. Find a behavior that is fun for you. Enjoy this—don't make it work. Play! Have fun with it. Consciously cultivate better NEAT habits. The mindfulness bell is an extremely powerful tool to use to consciously create new habits/routines. Use it! You can download it free for computers here: (http://bit.ly/1DQa53t), for android phones here: (http://bit.ly/1gWx4Cb), and for iPhones here: (http://apple.co/1wJL0Kz).

Move your body as constantly as possible throughout the day.

4. Then, and only then, worry about doing workouts

Once you are already standing the majority of the day and going for at least one walk each day, then and only then should you be worried about doing intense workouts. Once you have the foundation, you can add in intense workouts several times per week, such as sprinting or resistance exercise. Note: I am not a big fan of "cardio" as I find much of the research around its health benefits to be somewhat questionable (see Dr. James O' Keefe's TED talk *Run For Your Life! At a comfortable pace, and not too far*). And the research is very clear that it does not have a significant impact on fat loss. A slow walk on a treadmill desk while you work every day is likely to offer much more profound health and fat loss benefits than jogging 5 miles three or four times a week. But as far as exercise goes, I favor a mix of occasional sprinting and resistance exercise on top of a foundation of daily standing and walking. I believe this to be the absolute most effective set of movement habits for optimal health, a fast metabolism, and an ultra-lean body. (If you want a fat loss exercise program that I have personally designed, see my recommended products page here: http://bit.ly/1Mb7NST). But always remember that simple, ultra-gentle movement throughout the day is the foundation, and is way more powerful than any workout program for both health and fat loss.

We're just beginning to fully understand the consequences of prolonged sitting throughout the day, but it now appears that this is a major factor that not only contributes to fat gain, but even more importantly, damages our cellular and metabolic health in shockingly profound ways in incredibly short periods of time. When the sun is up, our bodies are meant to be standing and moving. If you want optimal cellular health, a fast metabolism, and a lean body, make sure you stand up and *move* throughout the day. I've said it before, but I really want to drill this into your heads because so many people don't know this: Standing and moving throughout the day isn't just a nice supplementary strategy to get some extra calorie burning in—it's a *requirement* for *normal* healthy cellular and metabolic function. It is as vital to cellular and metabolic health as food, water, and oxygen. For those of you who spend hours sitting every day, making this shift can be life-transforming.

In the words of Dr. Levine, "There should never be an hour that you're sitting down. Because your body idles. The gunk builds up. The blood sugar level rises. Blood fats elevate. In order to keep the fuels moving through the system (i.e. keep your metabolism running) you need to be moving every hour."[148]

---

148 BBC Documentary. The Truth About Exercise.

The Simple Nutrition Blueprint for Eliminating All the Nutritional Causes of Fat Gain

At this point you might be thinking, "Okay, well so what *exactly* am I supposed to eat?"

In this chapter, I'm going to provide you with an unbelievably simple blueprint to eliminate every single one of the nutritional factors that prevent your body fat set-point system from working to keep you effortlessly lean. This solution is so simple you're probably not going to believe that it could possibly eliminate every single one of these causes of fat gain. But I assure you, this simple blueprint is extremely powerful—*if* you make the commitment to follow it.

First, let me tell you what it *does not involve*:

- I'm NOT asking you to forcibly deprive your body of calories.
- I'm NOT asking you to forcibly restrict portion sizes.
- I'm NOT asking you to live la vida low-carb.
- I'm NOT asking you to eat low-fat.
- I'm NOT asking you to do some weird food combining diet.
- I'm NOT asking you to do intermittent fasting.

- I'm NOT asking you to eat every 2 hours or eat every 5 hours or not eat after 6pm or any other such arbitrary food timing pseudoscientific nonsense.
- I'm NOT asking you to deny and fight against your cravings.
- Most importantly, I'm NOT asking you to forcibly starve yourself through hunger!

Now, you're probably thinking, "There's no way you can show me a strategy that causes fat loss without forcibly restricting calories, portion sizes, eating low-carb, fasting, fighting your cravings, and fighting against hunger! Impossible!"

Not only am I going to show you a strategy that does all that, but it's also really the *only* way to achieve long-term *lasting* fat loss. In other words, anyone that you know that has achieved lasting fat loss hasn't done it because of their "calorie counting" or "low-carb" or "low-fat" diet (even though you and they might think so). In reality, it's because they unknowingly removed the causes of body fat set-point system dysfunction.

So what is the way to accomplish all this?

Simple: I want you to eat meals composed of whole-foods, with a focus on plant foods (fruits and vegetables especially) and protein-rich foods.

It's literally as simple as this:

- Step 1: Choose Your Protein(s): Beef, Chicken, Fish, Shrimp, Yogurt, Eggs, etc. (Vegans and vegetarians can use vegan protein sources to increase their protein intake).
- Step 2: Choose Your Fruit: Pineapple, Mangoes, Oranges, Pears, Blueberries, etc. (Yes, you can eat sugary fruits, not just blueberries).
- Step 3: Choose Your Vegetable(s): Potatoes, Lettuce, Kale, Carrots, Broccoli, Beets, Sweet Potatoes, Squash, Cabbage, etc. (Yes, you can eat starchy vegetables, not just salads.)

- Optional: Add in legumes/grains/nuts/seeds according to personal preference (preferably soaking and/or sprouting them).

Done. Meal created.

Above all else, make sure that every meal you eat consists of protein-rich foods and some fruits and/or vegetables.

That's it. And just with that one simple rule you can cause rapid, lasting, and effortless fat loss without suffering through hunger, macronutrient restriction (low-fat, low-carb etc.), or forcible calorie deprivation. That's literally all it takes.

This is about as effortless as it gets. You do have to do *something*. I am not going to sell you on the idea that you can get whatever result you want while continuing to do everything exactly as you currently do it. If you want a different result, you of course, have to change what you're doing. Having said that, this approach is all about doing things that have the greatest impact with the least amount of effort and the least amount of suffering—things which are in harmony with your biology rather than things which ask you to fight against your biology. This is a way of eating that does not ask you to restrict calories or portion sizes, or carbs or fat, or fight your cravings. Moreover, unlike some other notable diet gurus who oppose calorie counting, I am not telling you to eat nothing but protein, water, and fiber. (Yes, there are literally people out there preaching "diets don't work, but go on my diet of nothing but protein, fiber, and water"). Well, yeah, if you eat nothing but protein, water, and fiber (i.e. very little fat or carbohydrates—the major fuel sources of your cells, and the place where all normal humans get the bulk of their calories), it's virtually impossible to eat over 1,200 calories per day so of course you're going to lose weight. The problem is that you're not going to feel very good, you're going to be terribly fatigued, you're going to have to fight terrible cravings, and you'll cause yourself all sorts of hormonal dysfunction if you follow this way of eating for very long. Ultimately, it's about as sustainable as forced calorie deprivation—that is, it's *not* sustainable.

Now, something that is important to realize going into this is that eating this way will *not* cause fat loss as *fast* as starving yourself on calorie restriction diets. But, it will cause fat loss that actually lasts, and that's what really matters! A pound that comes off effortlessly stays off forever, a pound that you "work off" is going to eventually come back. Remember that.

This is not just another program that causes rapid, *short-term* weight loss, followed by a steady and unstoppable regaining of all that lost weight.

No, this program is different—this is the *real* solution to fat loss. This is the way to achieve lasting and sustainable fat loss—to achieve and maintain a lean body, effortlessly.

If you're focused on the speed of fat loss, consider that intelligence is highly correlated with long-term thinking, and lack of intelligence is correlated with short-term thinking. In other words, trying to approach fat loss by saying, "How can I lose 12 pounds this week?" or "How can I lose 30 pounds this month?" is the fool's way of approaching fat loss. (Note: If you want to do that, it's very easy to achieve. All you have to do is starve yourself—just eat 1,000 calories a day and work out. I guarantee you'll lose lots of weight, mostly from water and muscle, not fat, and then in six months, you'll be fatter than when you started.) The *intelligent* approach to fat loss is the one that asks, "How can I achieve fat loss in a way that is effortless (doesn't require willpower, deprivation, and suffering through hunger pangs), and achieve fat loss in a way that *lasts?*" That is the smart approach to fat loss.

In that sense, this guide is the intelligent person's blueprint to fat loss.

A quick note about carbs: This is NOT a low-carb diet! Many people see the recommendations to eat protein plus fruits and veggies, and in their minds, they immediately lump this nutrition plan in with low-carb Paleo type plans and come away thinking that I'm advocating a low-carb diet. No! I do not advocate low-carb diets. The diet I'm presenting here is *not* low-carb. To give you an idea of what I mean here, I personally eat 400-600g of carbohydrates each day—from fruits and root vegetables. Hardly low-carb. Many tribal populations around the world eat a diet that adheres to the template I'm presenting here and eat way *more* carbs than we do on the Standard American Diet (which is composed of just over 50% carbohydrate). To give you a few examples, the Kitavans eat a diet that's 69% carbohydrate—and all of their carbs come from fruit and starchy root vegetables. The Okinawans—a people world-renowned for their incredible longevity—eat a diet that is about 85% carbohydrate (mostly from sweet potatoes). And the Tukisenta people of New Guinea and the Ewe tribe in Africa eat a diet that is over 90% carbohydrate—they eat basically nothing but root vegetables all day long! By the way, if you're wondering, all of these tribes are extremely lean and virtually no incidences of people being overweight, let along obese. (It's worth checking out Guyenet's debunking of the Carbohydrate Hypothesis of Obesity if you haven't already). **Take away message: This is not a low-carb diet. Carbs are your friends, and you can eat them.**

(If you are eating a low-carb diet, you absolutely love it and you're one of those very rare people that actually functions best on a low-carb diet, by all means, continue doing it. But the vast majority of people that I've seen go low-carb don't accomplish anything except screwing up their metabolism and thyroid function).

Don't overthink this plan! I don't even want you to worry about which specific animal foods and which specific fruits and vegetables are the best choices. I don't want you to worry about trying to restrict fat or restrict carbs. I don't want you to feel restricted in any way. You can eat any animal proteins you want, any fruits you want, any vegetables you want. Whichever ones you enjoy and crave the most.

You want steak? Eat steak. You want chicken? Eat chicken. You want milk? Drink milk. You want potatoes? Eat potatoes. You want eggs? Eat eggs. You want mangoes? Eat mangoes.

Don't worry, "Oh, mangoes are a high sugar fruit," or "Potatoes have lots of carbs," or "Steak has saturated fat," or "Eggs have lots of cholesterol." Forget everything you think you know about nutrition, and for now, follow just one simple rule: **If it doesn't run, fly, swim or grow out of the ground, *don't eat it.***

Don't even worry about portion sizes or food timing. Eat according to *your biological need*. That means, eat how much your body craves. Eat *when* your body craves food (i.e. when you're hungry). And stop eating when you're full. Get back into harmony with your body, and get back into harmony with eating according to your body's biological need.

That's literally all you have to do.

Here's what I do not recommend eating on this program:

- **Anything processed.** You don't want foods in a package with ingredient lists. You want single-ingredient foods (i.e. "eggs," "oranges," "carrots," "blueberries," "halibut," etc.) not a packaged food with a long list of 20 different ingredients.

- **Large amounts of unsoaked/unsprouted grains—** both refined and unrefined grains. (Soaked and/or sprouted grains are perfectly acceptable, as long as you tolerate them).

- **Large amounts of unsoaked nuts and seeds** (and nut and seed oils/butters/milks), and legumes. (Soaked and/or sprouted seeds/nuts/legumes are perfectly acceptable, as long as you tolerate them).

- **Vegetable oils** (canola oil, safflower oil, corn oil, grape seed oil, soy oil, etc.).

Please note that I am not saying that these foods are poisons that will kill you, and you should never eat them. There's no need for this sort of extreme black-and-white reaction. You can still consume these foods in the amounts that are appropriate for you to feel that your diet is sustainable. I am simply telling you that these foods are not ideal sources of *any* nutrient and that you can get all needed nutrients from better sources. And I am recommending that you do just that!

If you absolutely cannot live some foods listed above and it stresses you out terribly to not have them in your life, by all means, carry on eating them. Whatever problematic compounds they have are probably less toxic than getting all stressed out over not being able to have them and then going on a binge.

You should never think about your food choices in the context of restriction. **The whole frame of restriction and forbidden foods is just wrong on every level. Your food choices should not be about avoiding calories, or fats, or carbs, or sugars or some specific list of "bad" foods. Your food choices should be about intentionally seeking out ideal sources of nutrients**. Instead of framing your dietary approach as "I must avoid so and so devil foods," frame it as "What are the best sources of nutrients and how can I focus more on eating those foods?" In other words, it's not about restricting yourself in any way—it's about progressively moving more and more towards the best sources of nutrients. The best sources of proteins, the best sources of fats, and the best sources of carbs/sugars. **Don't make your food choices focused on forcibly depriving yourself—make them about seeking out the best nutrients.** If you don't do that every single day or had a meal with processed junk food or just lower quality nutrients, you don't need to feel guilty about it. Relax. Breath. And in the future, make a point of seeking out better sources of nutrients that you know are giving your body what it needs. (We all need to find the appropriate balance that is sustainable for us--and that is going to be very different for each of us. Some of us may need regular indulgences while others do much better by indulging on only very rare occasions--and it's actually *easier for them,* since it eliminates chances of bingeing. This is a very individual thing.)

That's it. It's unbelievably simple, and I assure you it's also unbelievably powerful.

This way of eating provides ample proteins, carbs, and fats to your cells and is incredibly dense in metabolism-boosting micronutrients. It is, simply put, the most nutrient-dense diet you can possibly eat.

Again, this system isn't about trying to deprive your cells of nutrients, it's about trying to *give them all the best nutrients they need to function optimally.* It's fat loss through enhanced cell function, not by starving the cells.

This nutrition blueprint is ultimately about this underlying goal: Removing the factors in modern civilization that override your body fat set-point system and prevent it from doing its job of keeping you lean, and re-engaging the body fat set-point system so it can do its job effortlessly!

Simply put, if you *don't* remove these factors from your life, it is virtually *impossible* to get and *stay* lean over time. They will eventually win out and drive your body fat set-point up.

So your choice is pretty simple. You can either:

1. Get rid of all factors (processed food, high reward food, high food variety meals, disrupted circadian rhythm, excessive sitting and movement deficiency, etc.) in your life that prevent your body fat set-point system from working properly. Or ...

2. You can continue trying to rely on gym workouts and constant neurotic calorie counting, and the willpower to chronically force yourself to starve through hunger and resist neurological cravings in order to constantly ensure that you are not eating beyond your body's biological need. (And go through the suffering through hunger pangs, yo-yo dieting, and metabolism slowdown that goes with that approach.)

Those are your only options. There are really no other options when it comes to fat loss. My system is the alternative to the "fat loss by willpower and deprivation" model. **Either you can do it by re-engaging your biology and allowing it to work for you, or by constantly fighting against your biology.** You should be aware though, as I've explained previously, that over 95% of people who choose the fight-against-biology approach end up in total failure, regaining all the fat they lost within two years, and feeling utterly hopeless and defeated.

That's why I find the first option not only infinitely more effective and more intelligent, but also infinitely easier and less stressful.

On Balance and Sustainability

Please understand that there is no one-size-fits-all diet or lifestyle plan that works for everyone. We all have to find the balance that is appropriate for us as individuals.

If you absolutely can't live without cakes and Nutella, then you have to find ways of incorporating them into your life a way that allows you to have the foods you crave while also still getting the health and fat loss results you're after.

Each person has unique needs as an individual--which is influenced by their current lifestyle habits, their cultural upbringing, their personality, their goals, their subjective sense of what is difficult, and many other factors. We all have to understand that, and we all have to integrate new information into our lives accordingly. That is, we need to find the balance that is appropriate for us as *individuals*.

What I teach in this book are principles and ideal ways of going about things based on the science. From that understanding, each person has to customize those principles to their lifestyle, personality, and goals, and find the balance that is appropriate for them as individuals.

If a person who is currently obese and eating a diet of 95% processed junk food, just making the effort to have one more meal per week of whole foods is a great achievement. They certainly don't need to jump into eating nothing but whole foods.

If a person who is currently working a desk job can get an under desk cycle or make an effort to go for a 1-minute walk each hour, that's wonderful. They don't need to completely overhaul their lifestyle and do everything perfectly when it comes to NEAT.

If a person has terrible circadian rhythm habits, just taking the simple step of downloading f.lux on their computer (a free software that works automatically with no effort whatsoever) is a great step. There's no need to feel guilty about not being able to do *everything* right with circadian rhythm habits.

The book is a set of principles of what works to drive fat loss--it's not a one-size-fits-all program where everyone is *forced* to adhere to strict rules or be punished. It's not all-or-nothing, not black-or-white. It's simply a set of principles, and it's up to you to decide how far you want to move towards the ideal.

Your results are likely to parallel how much you move towards the ideal, but it's important to make sure you go about things sustainably and systematically rather than burning yourself out trying to do too much too quickly.

There are hundreds of thousands of people who eat 100% whole foods diets and find it perfectly easy and effortless to do so. There are also hundreds of thousands for whom eating a 100% whole foods diet would be completely tortuous and unsustainable. What is easy and effortless for one person is incredibly difficult for another. It's important for all of us to recognize that--particularly when it comes to diet and lifestyle change--and remember that it's up to all of us to integrate new information into our lives in a way that works for us as individuals.

To the extent that you can move towards the ideal, that's wonderful. To the extent that something is really difficult for you, that means you should back off and find the appropriate balance that works for you.

The goal is to find that perfect balance of changing your lifestyle habits enough to actually get fat loss results, but not try to go so extreme that it requires so much effort that it becomes unsustainable. Don't do so much that you can't sustain it, but do enough to create results. You don't have to do everything perfectly, but always be moving towards the ideal.

How You Should Eat

Below is a list of the different options you have in several different food categories. You can combine these in whatever way you like. It's very simple: All you have to do is pick something from each of the categories. Meal created. Done.

Step 1: Choose your preferred protein source from these foods:

- Eggs (ideally free-range)
- Dairy (Milk, Cheese, Yogurt, ideally pastured and raw/organic)
- Shellfish (ideally wild-caught)
- Fish (ideally wild-caught)
- Beef (ideally grass-fed)
- Wild Game Meats
- Lamb (ideally grass-fed)
- Turkey (ideally free-range)
- Chicken (ideally free-range)
- Pork (ideally pastured)
- Protein Powders (Whey, Casein, Egg, Vegan protein powders like Pea, Hemp, Potato, etc.)

NOTES: Ideally, choose organic and naturally-raised options. For vegans and vegetarians, I strongly recommend increasing protein consumption using vegan protein powders.

Step 2: Choose your preferred fruits and/or vegetables (and/or grains, legumes, nuts, and seeds):

FRUITS

- Citrus: Oranges, Grapefruits, Lemons, Limes, Tangerines, Mandarins, etc.
- Pineapples, Papayas, Mangoes, Kiwi Fruit, Grapes
- Berries: Blueberries, Raspberries, Blackberries, Strawberries, Cherries, etc.
- Apples, Pears, Pomegranates, Peaches, Plums, Nectarines
- Watermelon, Cantaloupe, Honeydew
- Superfruits such as Goji Berries, Acai Berries, etc.

VEGETABLES

- Potatoes, Sweet Potatoes, Yams, Yucca
- Spinach, Arugula, Romaine Lettuce and other Lettuce Varieties
- Carrots, Parsnips, Celery, Celery Root, Beets, Radishes
- Pumpkin, Butternut Squash, Yellow Squash, Zucchini
- Mushrooms (especially medicinal varieties such as Maitake, Shitake, etc.
- Cruciferous Vegetables such as Broccoli, Cabbage, Cauliflower, Brussels Sprouts, Kale
- Tomatoes, Avocados, Cucumbers, etc. (technically fruits but grouped here as vegetables to keep things simple)
- Onions, Garlic, Shallots, Peppers
- Herbs such as Basil, Cilantro, Parsley, Dill, etc.
- Sea Vegetables such as Nori, Kelp, Kombu, etc.

GRAINS/LEGUMES/NUTS/SEEDS

- Rice, Oats, Corn, Barley, Quinoa, etc
- Lentils and Beans

- Almonds, Cashews, Brazil Nuts, Macadamias, Chestnuts, Sunflower Seeds, Pumpkin Seeds, Chia seeds, Hemp seeds, etc.

(Because most health-conscious people are already eating large amounts of nuts/seeds/legumes/grains--or are generally familiar with eating them--the suggested meals in this book will focus more on fruits and vegetables as the base of meals. **I strongly recommend focusing meals around fruits and vegetables in preference to grains, legumes, and nuts/seeds.**)

NOTE: Yes, you can and should eat starchy vegetables like potatoes and yams. Yes, you can eat sugary fruits like mangoes and pineapples. You do not have to restrict carbs, but you DO want to get all your carbs from whole food sources.

A quick note on the above lists: These lists are obviously not meant to be all-inclusive—there are some proteins, fruits, vegetables, and other foods that are also acceptable, but they are not listed here. If they follow the principles outlined here, feel free to include them.

Cooking and Flavoring

1. The only cooking oils you should ever use are refined coconut oil or butter or ghee. No canola oil, corn oil, grapeseed oil, soy oil, safflower oil, sunflower oil, or others that are liquid at room temperature.

2. For sauces and dressings, do not use store-bought options because they're almost always packed with vegetable oils. Instead, make your own by using coconut oil/MCT oil, butter, ghee, olive oil, or yogurt as a base.

3. In general, you should get fats from whole foods rather than purified fats/oils. But as far as purified fats/oils go, you want to keep it limited to: Coconut oil, butter, ghee, MCT oil, and olive oil.

4. Use sea salt, herbs, spices, vinegars, and citrus juices according to your tastes for flavoring foods.

Drinking

1. Drink water as needed by your body when thirsty.
2. You may consume freshly made coffee and tea according to your taste.
3. Avoid soda (soda is processed, highly rewarding food).
4. Drink alcohol only in moderation, if at all (i.e. glass of wine a few times a week).

Eating Schedule

1. Eat when hungry. Eat only when hungry. Do not eat when not hungry. Stop eating when full. This is a very simple concept that we would all think of as obvious. Yet, virtually no one actually follows it and eats in accordance with the signals from their body. We have been taught endless ways of intellectually interfering with listening to our body's intelligence (e.g. don't eat how many calories your body wants, deny your cravings, don't eat after 6 pm even when hungry, eat every two hours even when not hungry, don't eat carbs, etc.). These will all screw you up in the long term. The best way to eat is in accordance with your instinctual needs just like every other creature on earth does. Sometimes the most powerful thing is also the simplest and most obvious.

2. In general, I recommend eating three meals per day and snacking in between meals only if necessary (i.e. if you are very hungry). I do not recommend this for any arbitrary reason as is so typical in the weight loss industry (e.g. "eat every two hours because it does such and such" or "eat five small meals per day" or "eat only two meals per day" or "don't eat after 6 pm"). I recommend it because this simple and normal schedule seems to be a fairly natural and universal eating schedule for humans around the world when they are in tune with their biological need for food. If you find that eating two meals a day works best for you, or five small meals seems most intuitive and natural for you, that's fine. However, in my experience,

most people do best when they eat breakfast, lunch, and dinner and snacks in between only if hungry.

3. Do not eat out of boredom. Do not eat to give yourself psychological pleasure. Eat only because of biological need, and get *in tune* with your biological need for food. Simple and obvious, but very powerful. It's not good enough just to understand this intellectually—you have to actually *do it*.

Sample Meals

If you still feel like you want to know *exactly* what to eat, below are sample meals for you to use. This is not meant to be a gourmet cookbook, but it will give you examples of some very simple (but tasty) and easy-to-prepare foods that meet all the criteria I've outlined in this book.

Note that some of the recipes below may mention terms like "free-range" or "organic" or "pastured" or "grass-fed" and in general, I do strongly recommend consuming foods (particularly animal foods) from naturally-raised environments. If you do not wish to do this because of either price differences or personal preference, feel free to disregard mention of these terms and choose conventionally raised versions of those foods.

These sample meals are not meant to limit you in any way, and you should feel free to create your own recipes that follow the guidelines above. Please note also that any listed **serving sizes are ultimately determined by your own biological need**. You should not be eating more than you need or forcibly eating less than you need. Remember, I cannot give you specific serving sizes that you force yourself to adhere to, as this is fundamentally at odds with you learning how to eat for your own biological need. The following sample meals are meant to show you what kind of meals you should be eating and to show you that you can still eat things that taste great on this eating plan.

One of the best aspects of this way of eating is that there are no complicated rules—no trying to count calories, figure out portion sizes, no figuring out percentages of fat, protein, carbohydrates, etc., no worrying about soluble vs. insoluble fiber, gluten vs. gluten-free, potential allergens in the diet, or high glycemic index vs. low glycemic index. Everything is taken care of by following the simple rule:

If it doesn't run, fly, swim, or grow out of the ground, *don't* eat it!

Eat only whole unrefined food. Each meal is composed of primarily animal proteins plus whole fruits and vegetables. Once you are eating a diet of mostly fruits, vegetables, and animal foods, then get into harmony with eating according to your biological need. Eat when you are hungry, don't eat when you're not hungry, and stop eating when you're full. If you have a craving for sugar, listen to the craving and eat the whole food source of that nutrient (eat fruit). If you have a craving for fat, listen to the craving and eat the whole food source of that nutrient (maybe some cheese). If you have a craving for salt, listen to the craving and eat the whole food source of that nutrient (maybe some potatoes sliced into fries and baked in the oven with a little coconut oil and a nice layer of salt). Your cravings are intelligent—work with the intelligence of your body by giving it what it craves, but give it the absolute best version of what it craves!

Having said that, here are some sample meals to use:

Breakfast

Hard Boiled Egg Mini Sandwiches: slices of hard boiled, free-range eggs, tomatoes, cucumbers, and avocado stacked on top of one another, seasoned with sea salt and pepper. Bowl of Fresh Fruit Salad.

Potato, Spinach, Mushroom, and Cheese Omelet: free-range eggs, spinach, mushrooms, potatoes, and organic cheese, seasoned with sea salt and pepper, and cooked in pastured butter or coconut oil. Bowl of Mixed Berries.

Blueberry Pineapple Parfait: plain organic yogurt, frozen blueberries, sliced bananas, chopped pineapple, shredded coconut flakes, and raisins.

Turkey and Egg Breakfast: free-range eggs scrambled in coconut oil or pastured butter, seasoned with sea salt and pepper and served with turkey sausage. Bowl of Fresh Pineapple with Chopped Mint Leaves.

Fruit and Protein Smoothie: fresh or frozen fruit, free-range egg whites, and/or whey/casein/egg/vegan protein powder, water or organic milk, and ice blended into a smoothie.

Yogurt and Fruit Compote: chopped apples, pears, and pitted dates cooked in a pot with cinnamon, lemon juice and a little water. Served warm over plain organic yogurt and sprinkled with shredded coconut flakes and more cinnamon.

Sunny Side Up Fiesta: free-range eggs cooked sunny side up in coconut oil or pastured butter. Topped with chopped tomatoes, avocado, corn, and cilantro, and seasoned with sea salt, pepper, and a squeeze of lime. **Bowl of Fresh Mango.**

Banana Milkshake and Mini Wraps: pastured organic milk, bananas, vanilla extract, and cinnamon all blended together into a shake. Slices of organic chicken breast and organic cheese rolled together into mini wraps.

Mediterranean Breakfast: free-range eggs cooked to your liking and topped with chopped cucumbers, tomatoes, avocado, and feta cheese. Seasoned with sea salt, pepper, olive oil, and lemon juice. Peaches and Tangerines.

Cheesy Scramble and Roasted Potatoes: free-range eggs scrambled in butter with organic cheddar cheese, seasoned with sea salt, pepper, and chopped chives. Served with roasted potato wedges. Oranges.

Italian Style Soft Boiled Eggs: soft boiled, free-range eggs with chopped tomatoes, basil, and shredded parmesan cheese, seasoned with sea salt, pepper, and a drizzle of olive oil. Bowl of Grapes.

Superfood Smoothie: bananas, goji berries, frozen blueberries, frozen blackberries, raw cacao powder, egg white, and/or whey/casein/egg/vegan protein powder, cinnamon, water, and ice blended into a smoothie.

Huevos Rancheros: free-range eggs cooked sunny side up in coconut oil, topped with tomato, avocado, jalapeno, onion, shredded cheese, and cilantro, seasoned with sea salt, and pepper. Bowl of Papaya with Lime Juice.

Coffee Milkshake and Goat Cheese Fruit Salad: bowl of fresh fruit salad topped with fresh mint leaves and organic goat cheese crumbles. Fresh coffee, organic milk, and raw honey blended into a shake.

Snacks

Bliss in a Bowl: frozen blueberries topped with plain organic yogurt, raw cacao nibs, coconut flakes, and cinnamon.

Goat Milk Yogurt & Berries: plain organic goat milk yogurt with raspberries, strawberries, lemon juice, and lemon zest.

Chocolate Cherry Shake: frozen cherries, raw cacao powder, egg whites and/or whey/casein/egg/vegan protein powder, ice, and water blended into a shake. Topped with raw cacao nibs.

Hard Boiled Eggs and Crunchy Carrots: hard-boiled eggs seasoned with sea salt and baby carrots.

Smoked Wild Salmon (Lox) and Cheese Mini Wraps: mini wraps made with wild Alaskan salmon (lox), organic cheese slices, sliced tomatoes, capers and chopped dill. Seasoned with pepper and lemon juice.

Beef Jerky and Oranges: home made organic, pastured beef jerky and oranges.

Steamed Shrimp & Mango Salsa: steamed wild-caught shrimp seasoned with sea salt and lime, dipped into mango salsa (chopped mangoes, red onion, cilantro, chili, lime juice, and salt).

Cheese and Grapes: organic cheese and grapes.

Simple Chocolate Mousse: plain organic yogurt, banana, raw cacao powder, and a pinch of sea salt, mixed in the blender and topped with fresh berries.

Lunch and Dinner

Halibut, Yams, and Mediterranean Salad: wild Alaskan halibut seasoned with herbs, sea salt and pepper, and baked in the oven. Served with baked yams and Mediterranean salad composed of chopped tomatoes, cucumbers, red onions, and organic feta chunks, seasoned with olive oil, lemon juice, sea salt and pepper.

Eggs with Root Vegetable Salad: soft-boiled or hard-boiled eggs served on a bed of salad greens topped with roasted root vegetables (carrots, parsnips, beets, radishes). Dressing made with plain organic yogurt, olive oil, lemon juice, fresh herbs, sea salt and pepper. Seasonal Fruit for Dessert.

Shrimp & Squash Skewers: grilled wild-caught shrimp and squash skewers with lime cilantro butter (melted pastured butter, lime juice, chopped cilantro, sea salt and pepper). Salad made with spinach, arugula, cilantro leaves, cherry tomatoes, avocado, radishes, and boiled purple potatoes. Simple salad dressing made with olive oil, lime juice, sea salt and pepper. Grilled Mangoes for Dessert.

Tuna & Sweet Potato Mash: wild-caught tuna fillet pan seared in coconut oil, served with sweet potato mash, sautéed shitake mushrooms and bok choy, all seasoned with sea salt and pepper.

Lamb and Roasted Vegetables: free-range lamb chops seasoned with sea salt, cayenne and black pepper, and sautéed in coconut oil. Served with roasted carrots, parsnips, cauliflower, onions, and garlic. Sauce made in the blender with plain organic yogurt, mint leaves, lemon, and salt.

Cod with Beet & Goat Cheese Salad: sautéed wild-caught cod seasoned with thyme, parsley, lemon, sea salt and pepper. Served with salad made of arugula, roasted yellow and red beets, and goat cheese. Strawberries for Dessert.

Chicken & Butternut Squash: organic free-range chicken seasoned with rosemary, garlic, lemon, sea salt and pepper, and roasted in the oven. Served with fork-mashed butternut squash and mushrooms sautéed in butter.

Baked Eggs & Boiled Yucca: free-range eggs baked in tomato sauce (made by blending tomatoes, fresh basil leaves, garlic, sea salt and red pepper flakes). Topped with grated Parmesan cheese and served with boiled yucca with garlic and an arugula salad with thinly sliced fennel, seasoned with lemon juice, olive oil, sea salt and pepper.

Scallops & Carrot Ginger Mash: wild-caught scallops sautéed in coconut oil, seasoned with lemon juice, sea salt and pepper and served over carrot and ginger mash and steamed spinach, seasoned with sea salt and pepper. Sliced Pears for Dessert.

Burger & Fries: burger patty made with grass-fed ground beef, sautéed onions and garlic, and chopped parsley. Seasoned with sea salt and pepper and grilled or sautéed to your desired doneness and then topped with organic cheese and served with oven roasted potato fries and tomato salad.

Steak with Herbed Potatoes: grilled grass-fed steak with herbed roasted potatoes and salad made of tomato, avocado, and shredded carrots. Dressing made of lemon juice, coconut oil, sea salt and pepper.

Chicken Soup: home-made chicken soup, made with organic free-range chicken, onions, garlic, carrots, celery, potatoes, and herbs, seasoned with sea salt, pepper and a good squeeze of lemon or lime.

Flounder with Creamy Polenta: wild-caught flounder fillet sautéed in butter with capers, shallots, cherry tomatoes, and basil. Served over creamy organic polenta.

Coconut Shrimp Curry: wild-caught shrimp, green onions, jalapeno peppers, red peppers, broccoli, and celery. All sautéed in coconut oil and then seasoned with curry seasoning, sea salt, pepper, fresh chopped cilantro, and a squeeze of lime. Served over white rice with shredded coconut flakes.

Clams, Mussels & Potato Wedges: clams and mussels steamed with shallots, cherry tomatoes, lemon juice, sea salt and pepper. Served with crispy, oven roasted potato wedges. Fruit Salad for Dessert.

Please note that some of meals may be more satiating than others. Simple dessert suggestions have been included in some of these sample meals, and not in others. This is *not* meant to say that you *must* have dessert if you eat that meal. Always eat according to biological need—without forcibly eating less or more than you need. Again, these sample meals are meant to give you an idea of how to eat this way, and to show you that eating this way doesn't need to be bland—these meals are *very tasty*.

Of course, in the modern world, we like to go out to eat with friends, and we don't always eat at the best places. In some restaurants, it may not even be possible to get a meal that is composed of whole foods cooked in good oils. I am human, and even I go out to eat at restaurants that are not ideal every once in a while. If you do go out to eat, just try to go to places where you can get very high quality foods. It's definitely doable. Even at places like Chipotle, you can get a meal of very high quality food that mostly adheres to the principles I've laid out here—and cheaply at that! So this is not exactly extreme. But for some people, it will require a change in habits, which can be uncomfortable at first. If you are in a situation where you absolutely must go to a low quality restaurant and you have absolutely no choice about it, it's not a huge deal if this happens once in a while. Again, these are exceptions to the rule I'm talking about here. In general, I would suggest finding a way to eat very high-quality whole foods, and before you start making exceptions here and there, I strongly suggest you build a foundation of the right habits—the most important being to break your addiction to processed foods, if you are currently addicted. Before dabbling in the world of cake and ice cream, make sure that you're eating a diet that is upwards of 95% pure whole foods the rest of the time.

But in general, I strongly recommend that you prioritize your life to make your own food at home as much as possible. This way of eating is very simple, but it does involve making the commitment to buy and prepare your own whole food and to get processed foods completely out of your diet. It doesn't have to be complicated gourmet recipes—just simple meals. For some of you, this may seem like a struggle at first, but I assure you, it can be done with minimal amounts of time and effort. And the reward of doing this is so great. Perhaps the single greatest predictor of leanness is the extent to which a person eats whole-food meals prepared at home. And the single greatest predictor of being overweight is not doing so.

If you want a different result than the one you're currently getting, you do have to do *something* differently. What I am presenting here is simply the least restrictive, most intelligent, and most efficient way of getting better results in your health and your body.

A Summary of the Golden Rules of Effortless and Lasting Fat Loss

1. **The High Food Reward Fix**: If it doesn't run, fly, swim, or grow out of the ground, stay away from it. Eat only whole unprocessed foods. Get over food addiction by giving in to your cravings rather than trying to fight them—but satisfy those cravings using the best quality versions of those nutrients.

2. **The High Food Variety Fix**: Eliminate calorie overconsumption by eating simple meals, not four-course meals or meals with a huge variety of different entrees, appetizers, sauces, etc.

3. **The Circadian Rhythm Fix:** Get lots of light during the day—particularly in the morning before noon. Eliminate or greatly reduce light in the blue spectrum after sunset. Supplement with micronutrients that most of us are deficient in, and which are linked to poor sleep. Sleep in complete darkness.

4. **The Fix for the Metabolic Toxicity of Chronic Calorie Overconsumption**: First, make sure you're following the above three recommendations. In addition, learn how to eat in accordance with your biological need (see #6 below), correct micronutrient deficiencies (see #8 below), and keep sitting to a minimum (see #9), since all of these will disrupt your ability to eat the amount of food your body actually needs. Most importantly, eat a diet of only whole, unprocessed foods and

make your daily goal to hit the target of eating upwards of 1g of protein per pound of lean body mass (or 1g per pound of bodyweight).

5. **The Fix for Metabolically Toxic Foods:** Eliminate vegetable oils from your diet. Eliminate trans-fats and allergens from your diet. Minimize consumption of food and drinks from plastics and cans. If you suspect gluten intolerance, get tested and/or eat gluten-free. If you consume lots of grains, legumes, lentils, nuts, and seeds, it's a smart idea to learn how to prepare them with soaking and/or sprouting.

6. **The Fix for Metabolic Damage from Forced Calorie Deprivation**: Don't be a cardio junkie and chronic calorie counter. Eat *according to your biological need*. That means: Do *not* try to forcibly restrict calories below what your body is telling you it needs—when you are hungry, eat. Eat when you're hungry and *only* when you're hungry, not out of boredom or to give yourself pleasure. Eat the amount your body is telling you that you need, and *stop* eating when you're full.

7. **The Anti-Fad Diet Fix**: Eat a diet composed of ample carbohydrates, proteins, and fats. And get those nutrients from the best sources of food for each of those nutrients. Moreover, learn from the *true* factors at the heart of the successes behind these fad diets—higher intake of whole foods and higher intake of protein. These two things can be tremendous allies in your fat loss efforts, and hundreds of thousands of people have achieved lasting fat loss from those two factors alone.

8. **The Micronutrient Deficiency Fix**: Eat an ultra-micronutrient-rich diet. This means, eat a whole food diet with a foundation of lots of fruits and vegetables.

9. **The Sitting Fix**: Transition from sitting to standing during the majority of the day. Walk and move as much you can throughout the day. The most powerful option is to get a treadmill desk. Next best is a standing desk, with a daily walk or two. At the very least, get an under desk cycle and use it throughout the day. Once you

have that foundation (and only once you have that foundation) in place, you can consider doing workouts. Many people get this backwards and worry about their workouts while being largely sedentary the rest of the time. This is a big mistake. The foundation is standing (i.e. minimizing sitting) and moving throughout the day and doing one or two daily walks. This is actually *more* powerful than doing an hour workout four of five times per week. Focus on minimizing sitting from your life and moving throughout the day. This strategy is incredibly powerful for those who currently work desk jobs. Sitting all day will completely sabotage your fat loss efforts. Standing and moving most of the day is a requirement for a healthy metabolism.

By following this simple set of strategies I've laid out here, you can eliminate and reverse every single factor linked to fat gain. These strategies will both spontaneously reduce calories-in and dramatically increase calories-out, which is how they work to create lasting and effortless fat loss. The key, however, is that they are doing this *without* any need for conscious forced calorie deprivation and suffering. They are doing it through enhanced cellular health! That means you are *not* just starving yourself into fat loss—you are actually sending your biology the signal to lower your body fat set-point!

No suffering through hunger pangs, cravings, fatigue, and the ravages of a reduced metabolic rate, which can result in a myriad of unwanted physical and mental declines. In fact, you should find yourself achieving fat loss, while feeling *more satisfied* with your meals, feeling *more* energetic, and actually *speeding up* your metabolism in the process.

That's fat loss by working with your biology, rather than against it!

Final Words

I assure you, this path to fat loss is not only infinitely more intelligent and more powerful than the typical mainstream approach of forced calorie deprivation. It's also a whole lot easier and doesn't cause any of the psychological suffering through hunger or fighting against cravings. So if you think what I'm advocating here is extreme or difficult to do, I suggest reframing your way of thinking about it, because what I've outlined here is basically the easiest, most effortless, least suffering-inducing, and most effective strategy ever created for lasting fat loss.

Finally, do not think of this as a "diet." This is a change in lifestyle—this is about aligning your lifestyle to be more in harmony with the environment in which your genes were shaped. It is a commitment to living in ways that are congruent with the needs of the human genome, so this is not something that you should think about in terms of "I'll do it for a couple months to try to lose weight." This is the single most powerful foundational step you can take to transform your body, as well as to fight against virtually every major degenerative disease that plagues western civilization today, from heart disease to cancer, diabetes, and countless others. This is the foundation for not only a great body, but also for your health and vitality for the rest of your life.

At the beginning of this book, I shared a simple quote with you:

"If a problem can be solved at all, to understand it and to know what to do about it are the same thing. On the other hand, doing something about a problem which you do not understand is like trying to clear away darkness by thrusting it aside with your hands."

As I've shown you in this book, the way that most people approach fat loss (calorie restriction and exercise) sets them up for failure because it doesn't really get at the real underlying biological factors that are driving fat gain in the first place.

In this book, I've debunked the Gluttony and Sloth paradigm of fat gain and the "eat less and burn more" approach to fat loss, and I've shown you the *real* factors driving fat gain and the obesity epidemic. That understanding is worth its weight in gold if you are trying to achieve fat loss.

Just as highly rewarding food, disrupted circadian rhythm, metabolic toxins, micronutrient deficiencies, forced calorie deprivation, fad diets, and sitting combine to create a state of physiology that drives *effortless fat gain,* so too does implementing the strategies in this book combine to create a state of physiology that drives *effortless fat loss.*

Ultimately, it is the difference between achieving fat loss effortlessly, or being one of the millions of people pursuing tortuous fat loss strategies that are getting them nowhere except thrown into a cycle of losing and regaining the same 10, 20 or 30 pounds over and over again, hopeless, defeated, and even fatter at the end of it all.

Fat loss is not about starvation and willpower—it's about *biology!* In this book, I've given you the blueprint to achieving fat loss by working with your biology instead of against it. And that, my friends, is the difference between failure and success.

Frequently Asked Questions

QUESTION: Did you encompass every factor that contributes to fat loss? What about _____?

There are several other factors that can sometimes contribute to fat gain and hinder fat loss. I will summarize them briefly here.

Psychological Stress: For some people, chronic psychological/emotional stress can be crippling to fat loss progress, so take steps to get this handled. Psychological stress can be a big one, and I strongly recommend making de-stressing a priority in your life if this is the case for you. Cognitive behavioral techniques, meditation, yoga, psychotherapy, walking in nature daily, breathing practices, making time for hobbies you're passionate about, reading, watching movies, laughing, and warm baths can all be powerful tools for de-stressing. Find the tools that work for your personality and temperament, and engage in them daily.

Hypothyroidism: Hypothyroidism is a major cause of fat gain—particularly in women in their 30s-50s. Thyroid hormone is the main regulator of metabolic rate, so naturally hypothyroidism almost leads to fat gain. In general, the state of physiology that typically goes with hypothyroidism–things like decreased sex/youth hormones, increased stress hormones, decreased blood flow to body fat tissues, decreased adrenoreceptor activity on body fat stores, etc—essentially prime the body for fat storage, and make it virtually impossible to lose fat. Correcting all of these (often complex) hormonal issues is beyond the scope of this book. But this is my area of specialty, and I have developed a program specifically for those with hypothyroidism and slow metabolisms to rejuvenate their metabolism and hormonal function. The strategies I presented in this book are the foundation for all my more advanced work with my hypothyroid clients, and once they are implementing everything contained in this book, my Metabolism Supercharge Program can step things up several notches.

Genetic diseases: There are certain extremely rare genetic conditions that essentially make you obese without there being a whole lot you can do about it. Fortunately, these conditions are exceedingly rare, and it's likely that no one reading this has one of these conditions. Even if so, it is likely that the strategies presented in this book could—at the very least—dramatically slow down the rate of fat gain.

Indoor Temperature Regulation: There is now some research indicating that chronically being indoors in temperature-regulated environments may be a factor that causes increased bodyfat set-point. Both exposure to very warm temperatures (saunas, exercise, hot baths) and exposure to cold temperatures (which help activate brown adipose tissue) are linked with metabolic benefits. Regularly spending time outdoors in nature and occasionally getting cold and getting very hot are likely good ideas for general health and, possibly, fat loss.

Meal Timing: Most of the research into the effects of meal timing on metabolic rate and calorie expenditure has shown minimal effects. The most famous of these meal timing myths that I'm referring to is of course the myth that "eating small meals every two hours will boost your metabolism relative to eating three big meals." Repeated studies have shown this to be false— that this sort of meal timing manipulation does not result in any more fat loss when matched for calories. Having said that, it may turn out that certain things, like skipping breakfast, for example (which is a habit associated with obesity), may in fact be a significant contributor to increased body fat set-point.

Metabolism Slowdown due to Old Age: I did not specifically address the metabolism slowdown that comes with aging. However, this isn't all that much different from all the sources of metabolic damage that I do talk about in the book. The metabolism slowdown that occurs with aging is generally a result of progressive mitochondrial dysfunction that is driven by a progressive accumulation of all the factors I did go over in this book. Thus, regardless of the source of that metabolic damage (i.e. aging, chronic sitting, chronic cardio, calorie and carb restriction, stress, lack of sleep, etc.), all of the strategies I recommend in the book are the foundation for rejuvenating the metabolism. The strategies in this book work just as powerfully for those in old age as they do for those who are young.

Gut Microbiome: There is evidence that the bacteria in our intestines may exert a profound influence on our body fatness. Research in this area is still developing, and it may eventually lead to key insights into obesity. Having said that, there is also evidence that one's diet exerts a profound influence on the gut microbiome, and that simply eating a whole-foods diet--rather than say, probiotics--may in fact be the most powerful way to fix an obesity-promoting gut microbiome.

Menopause: I didn't get into menopause in this book for a couple of reasons: First, it is an extremely controversial and contentious area that is hotly debated issue among scientists. There is no scientific consensus about the effects of estrogen. To give you an idea of what I mean, I could literally quote top experts on menopause and estrogen replacement therapy that say completely opposite things— one expert saying estrogen therapy is very healthy, another saying estrogen therapy will give you cancer and a whole bunch of other problems. One expert saying estrogen goes down after menopause, another expert saying that only blood estrogen goes down, but tissue concentration of estrogen actually *increases*. The truth is, there is no scientific consensus on menopause, what it does to the body, or what to do about it—even among scientists and physicians who specialize in that field. I don't think anyone knows it all when it comes to menopause and estrogen—and I am certainly not going to claim that I do. Second, it is such a complex topic that it would require a whole 200-page book in and of itself. And even then, some experts would completely disagree with everything I said. But yes, menopause can certainly change things very significantly. Like with aging, all of the strategies presented in this book will greatly help support metabolic health regardless of your age or menopause status.

Chemicals: Pesticides and other chemicals used in conventional farming, as well as plastic softeners like BPA, are now being linked to various hormonal issues in many animal species, including humans. It's too early to conclusively say that this is a factor driving fat gain, but in general, I do think it's a good idea to eat organic and eat/drink out of glass rather than plastic containers.

Prescription Drugs: There are several prescription drugs that create side effects that can result in fat gain over time—either as a result of fatigue or through promoting hormonal imbalance. This is a complex area and is beyond the scope of this book, but if you are taking prescription drugs, it is worth doing some research to figure out if that drug may be affecting your hormonal and metabolic function in such a way that promotes fat gain. If so, find another doctor and get a second opinion about whether it is absolutely necessary for you to be on that drug, and, if not, take steps with your doctor to wean yourself off.

There are likely other potential factors that can contribute to fat gain in some people, but this book has addressed the main factors that are known to science.

QUESTION: How can I make sure I'm doing everything right?

Having an objective accounting of your daily behaviors is important for us humans, as we are notoriously unconscious and often just plain delusional in the self-accounting of our behaviors. In addition, repetition can be extremely helpful in integrating habit changes into our lives. So here is my simple and easy solution:

Print out the following checklist, post it on your refrigerator, and at the end of the day, go through it and check off everything you did that day. I recommend printing a stack of these so you can go through one a day until these habits become natural and effortless for you. (Note: This only works if you actually *do it*—just reading about it right now won't have this effect. You actually do have to print this out and check things off every day.)

The Forever Fat Loss Daily Checklist:

Score yourself on a scale of 1-10 (10 being best) for each one. Add up your scores, and commit to making progressive weekly improvements until you consistently score between 95-100 each day.

- **Food Reward Fix**: I ate only whole unprocessed foods today.

- **The High Food Variety Fix**: I ate simple meals today, with single-ingredient foods.

- **The Circadian Rhythm Fix**: I minimized/eliminated my exposure to blue light after sunset. I got ample sunlight during the daylight hours (particularly before noon). I took micronutrient supplements to help my sleep. I am about to sleep in a completely dark room.

- **The Fix for the Metabolic Toxicity of Chronic Calorie Overconsumption**: I ate only whole, unprocessed foods today, and I ate in accordance with the signals from my body telling me when it was hungry/full. I put emphasis on having a high protein intake of roughly 1g per pound of lean body mass.

- **The Fix for Metabolically Toxic Foods**: I ate no trans-fats, fried foods, BPA-rich food products, or vegetable oils today.

- • **The Fix for Metabolic Damage from Dieting**: Today I ate *according to my biological need*. I did not try to forcibly restrict calories below what my body was telling me it needs—when I was hungry, I ate. I ate food *only* when I was hungry, and I didn't eat because I was bored or just mindlessly trying to give myself pleasure. I ate the amount of food that I felt I needed, and I stopped eating when I was full.

- • **The Anti-Fad Diet Fix**: I did not try to eat low-fat or vegetarian or low-carb, thinking that by avoiding some macronutrient I was making myself healthier or helping myself achieve fat loss. I understand that none of the macronutrients are evil, and I resolve to rid myself of the previous anti-macronutrient dogmas I have subscribed to in the past. (Unless I am doing it for either medical or ethical reasons).

- • **The Micronutrient Deficiency Fix**: Today I ate an ultra-micronutrient-rich diet. This means I ate a whole food diet with a foundation of tons of fruits and vegetables.

- • **The Sitting Fix**: I avoided sitting as much as possible today. I stood up and moved my body almost constantly during all (or virtually all) of my working hours today and worked at my standing desk or treadmill desk. I also went for at least one walk, ideally in the sun and in nature.

- • **Today I did absolutely everything I could to prioritize my cellular health—I ate ideal sources of nutrient-rich foods (where all of my meals consisted of high quality animal proteins plus fruits and/or vegetables), I took steps to ensure ideal circadian** rhythm function, and I made the effort to stand up and move my body for most of the day.

Free Test To Uncover the Hidden Factors Holding You Back From Losing Fat

In this book, I have debunked many of the myths and pseudoscience around fat loss, and showed you the real factors that determine your fat loss destiny.

As another tool that you can use in conjunction with this book, I have developed a special test (which is 100% *free*) that is designed specifically for the purpose of identifying which factors are holding you back from losing fat. The test will tally up your answers and give you a personalized result showing you what specific factors are holding you back from losing fat.

(Note: After taking the test, you will also be sent a free e-book- -*Unstuck: The 6 Potential Factors Sabotaging Your Fat Loss Efforts, and How to Fix Them.* This e-book is generally meant for those people who have *not* already read this book. It's simply a very short and less in-depth version of some of the information presented in *Forever Fat Loss* that talks about fat loss without going into all the details in this book. So please note it's **not necessary** to read that short e-book since you've already read this book).

Instead, here's what I suggest: **After taking the test and getting back your personalized results, you can then use those results to reference back to specific sections in this book that are relevant to the factors identified in the test. This will help give you more personalized guidance on specifically what factors you should be focusing on and allow you to approach your fat loss efforts in the most efficient way possible.**

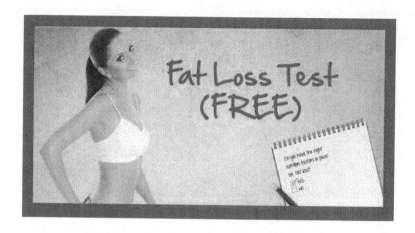

Take the test here: www.ariwhitten.com

One Small Request

The information in this book can change the paradigm in the fat loss industry, and can show people a real path to sustainable leanness. It can potentially help prevent millions of people from going on starvation diets and spinning their wheels, torturing themselves while achieving nothing but worse health and an even slower metabolism. But in order to do that, this information has to reach more people, and that depends on you! So please do me a big favor and write a review on this book. The more 5-star reviews it gets, the more this information will help others just like you escape from the dieting trap and transform their lives. Thank you so much for reading my book. I sincerely hope you will use this information to transform your life. I also hope you will leave a review and help others do the same. I greatly appreciate the time and effort you put into writing thoughtful reviews!

About the Author

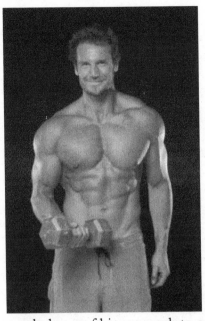

Ari Whitten is the #1 bestselling author of the cutting-edge book, *Forever Fat Loss*. He is a fat loss and nutrition expert who has been running a nutrition counseling and personal training business for over a decade. Ari has a Bachelor's of Science from San Diego State University in Kinesiology with a specialization in fitness, nutrition, and health. He holds two advanced certifications from the National Academy of Sports Medicine and recently completed coursework for his PhD in Clinical Psychology, an education which rounds out all aspects--nutrition, fitness, and psychology--of his approach to optimal health.

Ari is a tireless researcher who has obsessively devoted the last two decades of his life to the pursuit of being on the cutting-edge of the science on health, fitness, and nutrition. Ari's work is geared toward one purpose: To get effortless and permanent fat loss by working with your biology, rather than the painful and temporary fat loss one gets through programs that work against your biology. That is the focus of this book, as well as Ari's more advanced programs, such as *The Metabolism Supercharge* program (which is designed specifically for those with metabolic dysfunction and thyroid issues) and *The Forever Fat Loss Formula*. His other programs can be found on his website (www.ariwhitten.com).

The future of fat loss has arrived, and it's no longer about deprivation and willpower--it's about *biology*! Stop trying to fight against your biology and start working *with* your biology.

76669517R00115

Made in the USA
Columbia, SC
08 September 2017